DIGITAL
CONNECTION
IN HEALTH AND
SOCIAL WORK

PERSPECTIVES FROM COVID-19

T0093804

Other books you may be interested in:

Social Work and Covid-19: Lessons for Education and Practice
Edited by Denise Turner   9781913453619

Out of the Shadows: The Role of Social Workers in Disasters
Edited by Angie Bartoli, Maris Stratulis and Rebekah Pierre   9781915080073

*The Anti-racist Social Worker: Stories of Activism by Social Care
and Allied Health Professionals*
Edited by Tanya Moore and Glory Simango   9781914171413

Anti-racism in Social Work Practice
Edited by Angie Bartoli   9781909330139

To order, or for details of our bulk discounts, please go to our website
www.criticalpublishing.com or contact our distributor, Ingram Publisher Services
(IPS UK), 10 Thornbury Road, Plymouth PL6 7PP, telephone 01752 202301 or
email IPSUK.orders@ingramcontent.com.

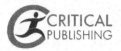

DIGITAL
CONNECTION
IN HEALTH AND
SOCIAL WORK

PERSPECTIVES FROM COVID-19

EDITED BY
DENISE TURNER AND MICHAEL FANNER

First published in 2022 by Critical Publishing Ltd

All rights reserved. No part of this publication may be reproduced, stored in a retrieval system, or transmitted in any form or by any means, electronic, mechanical, photocopying, recording or otherwise, without prior permission in writing from the publisher.

Copyright © 2022 Dr Denise Turner and Dr Michael Fanner

British Library Cataloguing in Publication Data
A CIP record for this book is available from the British Library

ISBN: 978-1-914171-92-5

This book is also available in the following e-book formats:
EPUB ISBN: 978-1-914171-93-2
Adobe e-book ISBN: 978-1-914171-94-9

The rights of Denise Turner and Michael Fanner to be identified as the Authors of this work have been asserted by them in accordance with the Copyright, Design and Patents Act 1988.

Cover design by Out of House Ltd
Text design by Greensplash
Project management by Newgen Publishing UK

Critical Publishing
3 Connaught Road
St Albans
AL3 5RX

www.criticalpublishing.com

Contents

Meet the authors

Dr Denise Turner is an experienced practitioner, registered social worker and academic. Prior to the pandemic she had already understood the importance of digital technologies for social work education and was chair of the advisory group for the national digital capabilities project for social work, commissioned by Health Education England and delivered by the Social Care Institute for Excellence and British Association of Social Workers (BASW). Denise's research has focused on varying aspects of digital practices, including a study on social workers' experiences of using technology in the assessed and supported year in employment. She is published on her research and development work and has also sole edited a previous book on the pandemic – *Social Work and Covid-19: Lessons for Education and Practice*. Denise is associate editor for continuing professional development for the journal *Child Abuse Review*.

Dr Michael Fanner graduated as an Adult Nurse (2012) and a Specialist Community Public Health Nurse/Health Visitor (2013) at King's College London/ He was awarded a PhD in critical social policy at the University of Greenwich in 2020. Up until 2018, Michael worked in a variety of clinical, academic and voluntary organisations in child protection, health visiting and emergency care. In 2018, Michael became a lecturer at the University of West London and was a main architect of the UK's first MSc Paramedic Science (Pre-registration) and subsequent module leader and teacher for the population health and behavioural science, evidence translation, dissertation and complex paramedic care delivery modules. Since 2021, Michael has been a Senior Lecturer in Specialist Community Public Health Nursing at the University of Hertfordshire and leads on the safeguarding, research methods, public health and social policy modules and is also a second supervisor on two doctoral research projects. Michael has research interests in how ethically complex social issues are 'dealt with' in clinical practice. Michael is an Associate Editor for *Child Abuse Review* and is also a Board Member at Bournemouth and Poole College. In his spare time, he volunteers for St John Ambulance.

Michaela Dunn is a Lecturer in Social Work at Goldsmiths, University of London. She previously held varied social work roles, empowering and helping children, young people and families across a spectrum of social care services, both statutory and voluntary sectors. She has learning and development interests centring on leadership, the interaction, exchange, and curiosity of personal and professional identities, and creative social work practices. She is also the Goldsmiths Academic and Evaluation Lead for the New Town Culture Project.

Dr Sandra Engstrom has a BA(H) in Sociology from Acadia University, bachelor and master's degrees in social work (specialising in leadership in international social work) from the University of Calgary and completed her PhD from the University of Edinburgh. She has practice experience with youth in Canada, Vanuatu, England, St Lucia and Scotland. She has worked with older populations in Florida and has volunteered with HIV organisations in Canada, Vanuatu, St Lucia, England and Scotland. She currently volunteers her time with the Stirling Rowing Club and Riverside Community Council. Her research centres on community resilience as well as the role of social work in combating the climate crisis. This often takes the form of looking at community mental health, trauma and eco-grief. Sandra has experience working with vulnerable populations as well as community groups within a research and teaching capacity. She primarily works within interdisciplinary settings and works with ecologists, health psychologists, public health, geographers, sociologists, anthropologists and archaeologists. Sandra works within the umbrella of qualitative methods and has experience with focus groups, in-depth interviews, photo-voice and autoethnography. When not working, you can find her out in the hills, on a river, or in a yoga studio.

Professor David T Evans, OBE, National Teaching Fellow, is Professor in Sexualities and Genders: Health and Well-being at the University of Greenwich. He is a registered nurse and teacher and has taught health and social care staff, in the UK and sometimes abroad, since 1990. His main publications are listed on his Researchgate profile (www.researchgate.net/profile/David-Evans-48/publications), with conference publications and CV at https://davidtevans.wordpress.com. David is experienced in andragogic e-learning provision and an active member of his wider University of Greenwich digital community.

Craig Harman has worked in the NHS ambulance sector for nearly 20 years, in London and in Scotland. In 2019 Craig took on the national role of Director of Health Operations at St John Ambulance in England, responsible for 30,000 St John people who work and volunteer in your communities. Craig is also an NHS Assembly member, advising the board of NHS England and Improvement about the Long Term Plan.

Annie Ho gained her qualification as a social worker in 1989, since when she has been working in local authority adult social care. Her specialist areas of work, knowledge and experience have been in the Mental Capacity Act, deprivation of liberty safeguards and safeguarding adults. She currently works as a principal social worker for adults and volunteers as a coach for BASW professional support services and as a spiritual accompanier and an Anna Friend (ministry for older people) for the Church of England. Annie is a qualified best interests assessor and continues to enjoy one-to-one work with vulnerable adults. She leads on work for her local authority on the workforce race equality standards for social care, piloting this as one of 17 local authorities selected by the Department of Health and Social Care. Annie is passionate about value-based and rights-based social work, and the equalities agenda is a key element of all her work. Together with maintaining her professional development in social work and leadership training, she completed an MA in fine art in 2015 and continues to develop her practice in art. She enjoys exploring the synergies between the professional discipline of social work and the creative opportunities offered by spirituality and art.

Barbara Hoyle began her career as a registered nurse in 1976 at Bart's Hospital and went on to train as a midwife and then a health visitor. In 2002 she was enrolled by NHS North West to become one of the first practice placement facilitators and since then has worked as a senior lecturer at the University of Central Lancashire, became a senior manager in an NHS Trust leading on medical and non-medical education, and then in 2012 she worked for a year as a Voluntary Service Overseas volunteer with the Nurses and Midwives Council of Malawi on a post-registration action research project in collaboration with the University of Washington. On her return, Barbara joined the University of West London and in 2014 became Head of Practice Education until her retirement in June 2021.

Rachel Parry Hughes is a senior social worker in a local authority adult social care service and a social work practice educator. She previously worked as a lecturer in social work at Goldsmiths, University of London, where she carried out research into the New Town Culture programme, a collaboration between artists, curators and social workers in the London Borough of Barking and Dagenham. Rachel is the author of the report on this research: 'The New Town Culture programme 2018–2020: Art, Creativity and Care'. This report identified five key creative processes which characterise the programme. Rachel subsequently led on the design of a CPD strategy for social workers and social care workers aimed at embedding these creative processes within the culture of the local authority.

George Keal, MStJ, graduated in adult nursing from Kingston University and St George's University of London in 2017. George is also a third-year graduate entry medical student at the University of Southampton. Alongside his full-time studies, George works as an emergency department nurse at Salisbury District Hospital. In addition to his studies and professional work, George is a district clinical officer and event nurse for St John Ambulance. In recognition for his work towards training and clinical education during the pandemic, he was awarded Membership of the Order of St John in February 2021.

Timothy Kuhn is a Faculty of Intensive Care Medicine accredited advanced critical care practitioner. He is a nurse by background and has worked in the critical care environment since qualifying in 2008. During his time within the critical care field, Timothy has undertaken a number of different roles including clinical, education and management. As well as a number of clinical qualifications, he has completed a master's degree in trauma sciences and a postgraduate diploma in advanced critical care practice. His professional interests include clinical education, trauma, extracorporeal life support and clinical governance.

Andrew Linton completed his social work education at the University of Oxford. He commenced as Lecturer in social work at Goldsmiths, University of London in March 2020. Prior to that he has been involved in managing social work education programmes at a number of universities including London, Metropolitan University, Brunel University, the University of Greenwich and the University of Hertfordshire. Andrew is passionate about reforming and improving social work practice and he is keen to develop creative, developmental and inclusive approaches in his work. Andrew is keen to promote critical social work practice and education, which enables practitioners to engage with individuals with lived experience, in deeper, more nuanced and creative practice.

Henrietta Mbeah-Bankas is the Head of Blended Learning and the Digital Learning and Development Lead at Health Education England. She was previously the Topol Technology Review Project Lead and a Clinical Nursing Fellow (Research and Evaluation) at NHS England/Improvement. She is a Registered Mental Health Nurse, a Darzi Fellow Alumnus, and an NHS Clinical Entrepreneur. She was a visiting nursing lecturer at City University of London and is currently a visiting lecturer/honorary research assistant at University College London. Henrietta's research interest is on equitable access to healthcare, particularly for individuals from minority ethnic backgrounds. She has contributed to the development and publication of a variety of materials, including policy and guidance documents in healthcare education and service delivery, journal publications, and nursing regulatory standards. She has an eclectic background but is currently focusing on the development of digital capabilities and the use of digital technologies in educating and training the health and care workforce.

Natalie Ravenscroft is the Wellbeing Support Manager and joined the National Activity Providers Association (NAPA) in 2021. She is a well-being practitioner with many years' experience developing creative activity and well-being programmes for people with learning disabilities, older people and people living with dementia. She manages the NAPA activity Support Service;

this includes the Helpline service, Support forums and NAPA Calendar. She also oversee several projects and partnerships. In her spare time Natalie is a keen cook, seasonal decorator and Tudor fanatic. She spends her weekends with her family and friends and travelling. She has two sons who serve in the British Army, a husband and three dogs.

Hilary Woodhead is Executive Director of NAPA, joining the organisation in 2019. She leads the organisation and oversees all aspects of the charity's work. Her focus is on championing excellence in activity, arts and engagement, the well-being of those who use care support services and the professional development of the activity workforce. She is a national and international speaker and facilitator and has extensive knowledge and expertise across a wide range of care, support and NHS services. Prior to joining NAPA, Hilary was the Co-Director of Support In Dementia (SiD), a dementia specialist support agency providing project management and staff development programmes across the health, housing and social care sector. She has a BA (Hons) in The Arts (Drama) and MA in Social Work (Social Care Management). She is a qualified adult learning facilitator with a special interest in dementia, the arts and the concept of well-being. In her spare time she enjoys interior design, musicals and dachshunds. She lives in Brighton with her partner. She has three children plus a dog, a cat and a tortoise.

BASW students are the team behind the British Association of Social Workers (BASW) students Twitter account. They manage and maintain the Twitter account voluntarily and are all student members of BASW. The team consists of social work students from across the UK who came together virtually through the social media platform Twitter. They all shared a newfound interest in using social media, primarily through the Covid-19 pandemic, and had a collective desire to meet students from different parts of the UK. The BASW students Twitter account provides a central point for student BASW members from across the UK to discover everything that BASW has to offer, such as CPD, training, events and networking opportunities. It was from this initiative that they found friendships which would never have evolved if it wasn't for social media during Covid-19. The group have supported each other during their transition as part of the 'virtual generation' of student social workers.

Foreword

Mark Nicholas, Chief Social Worker for NHS Digital

Reading the reflections in this book on digital connection during the pandemic encouraged me to think about my own experience. At the beginning of March 2020, I was working as Chief Social Worker for NHS Digital with responsibilities for a range of digital systems, but little appreciation of being at the beginning of an international pandemic which would impact profoundly on the work we were doing. Over the subsequent months, the scope of my work grew from the nhs.uk website, the NHS App and our Social Care Programme to involvement in the vaccine rollout and Covid pass, while also working with colleagues to provide frontline health and social care workers with the digital tools they needed to do their jobs. This meant providing secure email and videoconferencing to care homes to allow sharing of information with the NHS, collecting data on infection rates and bed capacity in social care, and developing guidance for social workers on getting the best from working virtually, among many other things. Throughout this time, the issue of digital skills in social care cropped up again and again, and Chapter 5 captures some of this nicely. It was also inspirational to witness that the NHS and social care work best together when they value each other's perspectives, experience and training. In particular, the habit of reflective practice, instilled through social work training, was of significant value in learning the lessons from the crisis. These three themes – digital skills, professional cross-collaboration and reflective learning – run through many of the chapters in this book and I'm really grateful to the editors and contributors for putting them together.

Introducing the book

Digital Connection in Health and Social Work: Perspectives from Covid-19 brings together a collection of diverse authors, comprising educators, practitioners and students, who offer their individual and collective perspectives of working and studying during the first 18 months of the Covid-19 pandemic. The book is a companion volume to *Social Work and Covid-19: Lessons for Education and Practice* (Turner, 2021), which focused solely on social work responses to the early stages of the Covid-19 pandemic in the UK. This book extends that focus by including health responses and in this way reflects the multi-disciplinary nature of practice by combining distinct professional voices, including those of paramedics and care home activity providers.

As co-editors, we believe that one of the strengths of this book lies in combining the voices of practitioners who may encounter each other in the course of their working lives, but perhaps never have the time to pause and consider the nature of other professional experiences. This book helps to provide that pause by creating a space for reflection for those who have been immersed in the pandemic responses, together with a celebration of the breadth and scope of achievements across the sectors, and a sharing of emerging 'best practices' between health and social work education and practice. The focus of the book is on the digital connections forged out of necessity when the UK first entered lockdown in March 2020, mediating much of our professional and personal lives through the affordances of the internet, and the book provides various case study examples of digital connection which can be applied to multi-disciplinary learning and practice.

Relevance of the book

In the 2018 annual review of diseases, the World Health Organization (WHO) (2018) listed eight priority diseases including Zika disease, Crimean-Congo Haemorrhagic Fever and 'Disease X', which were considered as threatening public health emergencies to global health. Each priority disease is considered a public health emergency where there is no standardised, evidence-based or known solutions in terms of prevention, treatments or cures. In 2018, the WHO termed a new priority disease 'Disease X' as a placeholder name that, in short, represents a hypothetical, unknown pathogen with similarly unknown effects upon the human body capable of causing a pandemic. Disease X is, in effect, what the novel coronavirus discovered in 2019 in Wuhan, People's Republic of China was destined to become.

This virus, now so well known to us as Covid-19, has altered our social and professional connectivity in previously unparalleled ways, significantly embedding increased digitalisation at the hub of daily life. Large populations across the UK have been forced to acquire new skills and connect to previously unfamiliar and indeed unknown platforms, forcing practitioners and educators alike into new ways of learning and knowing, with a greater emphasis on co-producing responses with students and service users. Our digital competence has evolved but alongside this, so have many of the ethical challenges which accompany such rapid digitisation (Goldkind et al, 2020) alongside new health challenges – for example, children with long Covid – where research in the field is still emerging (Fanner and Maxwell, 2021).

In its Research and Development Blueprint for Action to Prevent Epidemics, the WHO (2018) aims to focus global efforts in research and development activities in order to reduce the time taken between the identification of an emerging outbreak and government approval of screening and diagnostic technologies, preventative and curative treatments and approaches for mass dissemination. This reduction in time hopes to prevent mass mortality and morbidity and avert public health crises, as well as planning for sufficient infrastructures (such as vaccine manufacturing facilities). The WHO articulates that as our world becomes more interconnected through rapid urbanisation, intensive farming practices, climate change, deforestation and globalisation, there are increased vulnerabilities for diseases to transmit via animals-to-humans and humans-to-humans alike. It is unlikely that any individual country or even region was ever truly prepared for the Covid-19 pandemic, but consequential international and government action has reflected the aims of the blueprint. Concomitantly, as the Covid-19 pandemic has graphically illustrated, the health crises have placed unparalleled pressures on the social work and social care sectors, with over 40,000 deaths in UK care homes (Sabin, 2021) and social workers dubbed the 'forgotten frontline' (BASW, 2021).

It is our hope as co-editors that the perspectives on living and working alongside Covid-19 offered in this book will prove useful in the future with the continuation of this current Covid-19 pandemic, as well as future outbreaks of new diseases predicted by the WHO across the globe.

Structure of the book

This book gathers perspectives from health and social work education and practice to illustrate different innovative ways in which online connectivity has been used positively to meet the multiple challenges of the pandemic. In this way the book acts as a valuable resource as we continue to meet the struggles of an existing global pandemic while simultaneously planning for the next. While this book is concerned with perspectives from health, social work and social care, we have purposively integrated the chapters to reflect the inter-connected nature of practice. Each chapter also ends with a set of reflective questions which can be applied to inter-disciplinary education and practice.

The first two parts of this book illustrate not only how those in the helping professions adapted and succeeded but also how connections were made possible in a variety of ways, including digitally. These first two parts offer ways of reimagining the traditional approaches used by educators and practitioners, by demonstrating how we can maximise the learner experience to be as 'workforce-ready' as possible, digitally – via remote, online, and virtual interactions – as well as by improving professional responses in responding to new challenges and uncertain times.

In the first chapter of **Perspectives from Higher Education, 'The trouble with normal': Covid-19's legacy and the multipotentiality for co-creating teaching, learning and assessing**, Professor David T Evans argues that the pandemic has challenged the more traditional ways of providing, teaching, learning and assessing, as well as reducing the possibilities for 'real' human-to-human contact – both in class and in professional or clinical practice settings. Drawing from multiple case examples, the chapter explores the potential of new methods and outlines suggestions for dealing constructively, positively and compassionately with barriers to a whole-system rethink for future directions, inclusive of institutions, teachers and learners.

In Chapter 2, **Reflecting on population health learning in pre-registration paramedic education during a global pandemic**, Dr Michael Fanner explores the rapid changes to paramedic education as a consequence of the pandemic. The chapter offers a brief history of the evolution and professionalisation of paramedic education, moving on to specific examples from the paramedic education curriculum. The chapter concludes with an exploration of recent literature on experiences of student paramedics across the globe. The chapter will be fascinating for many of those outside of the specific paramedic discipline who may still view those in the profession largely as 'ambulance drivers'.

In Chapter 3, **How Covid-19 has impacted upon the practice learning experience of pre-registration nursing students**, Barbara Hoyle describes the lived experience of trying to manage the practice learning requirements of pre-registration nursing students during the challenges of Covid-19. Echoing other chapters within the book, this chapter highlights the previously unprecedented challenges of transitioning to a new curriculum during this period, and the necessity of an accelerated technical shift in communication and learning approaches.

Chapter 3 was written from the perspective of a Head of Practice Education, and is complemented by the next contribution which is written by student social workers who were directly affected by changes to practice education and education during the pandemic. In Chapter 4, **Covid-19 and the virtual generation**, the student team who make up the British Association of Social Workers (BASW) Twitter account reflect on the impact of the pandemic on their individual and collective experiences of learning, access, well-being and placements during this time. The chapter is a testimony to the contributors' commitment to joining the social work profession at such a challenging time.

Chapter 5, **'I am not a cat': Digital capabilities and Covid-19**, written by Dr Denise Turner, resonates with other chapters in the book in exploring some of the significant digital opportunities as well as the challenges resulting from the Covid-19 pandemic via the three main domains of the Social Care Institute for Excellence (SCIE) and the British Association of Social Workers' (BASW) Digital Capabilities for Social Workers statement (SCIE and BASW, 2020). Reporting in March 2020 and thereby coinciding with the first national UK lockdown, this project commissioned by Health Education England produced several resources including a framework for the skills and values that social workers require in order to practise digitally with children and adults. The project echoes similar developments in health, where there has also been a shift to embedding digital technologies and which are similarly showcased throughout the book. The chapter takes its title from the viral video of a United States lawyer who, during a live court trial, was unable to remove the cat filter on his video call, thereby emphasising the importance of digital professionalism and capability.

Chapter 6, **Educating the future health workforce for the delivery of twenty-first-century care**, opens the next part, **Perspectives on Practice**. Written by Henrietta Mbeah-Bankas, who is head of blended learning and development for Health Education England and was a stakeholder in the Digital Capabilities for Social Work project described in Chapter 5, this chapter showcases the accelerated changes made by educators, health professional leaders, regulators and professional bodies to embed emerging innovative technologies in the health workforce. The chapter takes a positive stance towards developments in digital learning, including simulation, augmented and virtual reality and other more contemporary ways of monitoring engagement through data analytics. Crucially for the focus of this book, the chapter emphasises the necessity of collaboration between higher education providers and technology companies, meaningful consultation with staff and learners and a culture that is open to change, arguing for an accompanying move away from viewing online learning as 'second-rated education'.

Chapter 7, **Putting down the laptop and rolling up the sleeves: Mobilising a workforce of medical students to the Covid-19 frontline and its impact on their education**, combines themes from the preceding chapters and moves these into a prac-tice context as George Keal, a registered nurse, showcases his individual experience as a third-year graduate-entry medical student during the pandemic. From George's perspective, practice and learning are brought together graphically as he describes the changes made to his own education alongside the ways in which medical students were prepared for the frontline.

In Chapter 8, **Digitalising the volunteer workforce development to support NHS delivery during Covid-19**, Craig Harman describes a similar mobilisation of the frontline undertaken by St John Ambulance, so well-known to the public for pro-viding generations with vital first aid work and visible at many public functions. As the chapter highlights, within a day of the global pandemic being declared, St John Ambulance had launched its Pandemic National Plan, putting an emergency command and control structure in place to support the NHS and national communi-ties throughout the crisis. By 1 April 2020, all St John operations had been diverted to play a role in the national emergency, with unprecedented speed of response. As part of this response, the organisation also had to embrace digital transformation, a theme throughout all chapters in this book.

Mobilisation of the workforce in a similarly impressive manner is the central focus of Chapter 9, **Practice teaching experiences of preparing redeployed workforces for critical care during the Covid-19 pandemic**. The author, Timothy Kuhn, describes how the pandemic placed NHS critical care services under severe pressure, resulting in the expansion of provision and workforce numbers. Concomitantly, this resulted in a demand for upskilling of non-critical care clinical workforces to help treat ser-iously ill patients, alongside maintaining continuing professional development (CPD) for trained critical care staff. Like all the chapters in this book, the impressive contri-bution of health and social care in adapting to rapidly changing circumstances during the pandemic is clearly emphasised.

In the final part, **Perspectives on Environments, Creativity and Well-being**, this impressive adaptation continues as a theme in Chapter 10, authored by Hilary

Woodhead and Natalie Ravenscroft of the National Activity Providers Association (NAPA), which focuses on **Supporting care homes to be digitally connected**. The shocking impact of Covid-19 on the care home sector was widely reported in the media and this impressive contribution showcases how NAPA, a national charity and membership organisation, met the challenge by adopting a digital approach to support care homes in adapting to technology-based approaches and new ways of working during the Covid-19 pandemic. The chapter provides some moving case examples including the use of virtual reality to illuminate how technology was used to mitigate some of the profound isolation and trauma experienced by care home residents during the pandemic.

In Chapter 11, the theme of creativity is picked up by Michaela Dunn, Rachel Parry Hughes and Andrew Linton, three academics from Goldsmiths, University of London, in their chapter **Creative social work in a virtual world: A case study on a work-based learning module**. The chapter describes moving an inspirational arts-based practice learning module for social workers and social care practitioners online, thereby over-coming the challenges of retaining creativity and connection despite the often distan-cing impacts of the computer screen. The chapter carefully considers the practitioner viewpoint and their contribution to the module, exploring and expanding upon the inherent need for creativity in social work and how this may translate into practice.

Chapter 12, **Mindfulness, social work leadership and Covid-19**, written by artist and principal social worker Annie Ho, maintains the focus on creativity, with an explor-ation of mindfulness in personal and professional disciplines. The chapter offers a very personal account, written from the perspective of a principal social worker and manager, charting the experience of applying mindfulness during the Covid-19 pan-demic and combining this with creativity to maintain an attitude of curiosity, sensi-tivity and kindness in social work practice. As with all other chapters in the book, the chapter explores the ethical challenges accompanying the move to digital solutions in social work while also showcasing the opportunities.

The final chapter is perhaps one of the most important contributions moving for-ward, as Dr Sandra Engstrom poses the question **Can we keep the environment in mind while we adjust to renewed freedoms?** Beginning with the rapid move online during the first UK lockdown in March 2020, the chapter emphasises the posi-tive benefits of reduced fossil fuel consumption and other environmental benefits and offers the reader an opportunity to reflect on what positive environmental changes happened within their own personal and professional spheres. The chapter ends with the hope that some of these sustainable changes can be maintained as we move into an unprecedented era of climate crisis and potential pandemics.

It is with this chapter and its accompanying message of hope for sustainable change that the book closes. Each individual chapter and the book as a collective contribution emphasises how, beyond teaching and learning, the UK health and social work sectors have moved from immediate 'firefighting' to adapting services for online and blended delivery. While the immediacy of being physically present has often deprived educators, students, service users and practitioners alike of face-to-face contact, chapters in the book illuminate ways in which the pandemic has also generated possibilities for creative and innovative learning and practices while building online communities, saving money on expensive travel and mitigating damage to the environment.

References

British Association of Social Work (BASW) (2021) Survey unveils the heavy toll on social workers – a 'forgotten frontline' – as restrictions limit their capacity to safeguard vulnerable adults and children. [online] Available at: www.basw.co.uk/media/news/2021/jan/survey-unveils-heavy-toll-social-workers--'forgotten-frontline'--restrictions (accessed 12 November 2021).

Fanner, M and Maxwell, E (2021) Children with Long Covid: Co-producing a Specialist Community Public Health Nursing Response. *Journal of Health Visiting*, 9(10): 418–24.

Goldkind, L, LaMendola, W and Taylor-Beswick, A (2020) Tackling Covid-19 is a Crucible for Privacy. *Journal of Technology in Human Services*, 38(2): 89–90.

Sabin, L (2021) England's Covid care home deaths could be thousands higher than official figures, say providers. *The Independent.* [online] Available at: www.independent.co.uk/news/uk/home-news/covid-care-home-deaths-higher-b1894592.html (accessed 12 November 2021).

Social Care Institute for Excellence (SCIE) and British Association of Social Work (BASW) (2020) Digital Capabilities for Social Workers. [online] Available at: www.basw.co.uk/digital-capabilities-statement-social-workers (accessed 20 January 2022).

Turner, D (ed) (2021) *Social Work and Covid-19: Lessons for Education and Practice.* St Albans: Critical Publishing.

World Health Organization (WHO) (2018) Annual review of diseases prioritised under the Research and Development Blueprint. Informal consultation. 6–7 February. Geneva, Switzerland. Meeting report. [online] Available at: https://web.archive.org/web/20200609040339/http://origin.who.int/emergencies/diseases/2018prioritization-report.pdf (accessed 12 November 2021).

Part 1 | Perspectives from Higher Education

Chapter 1 | 'The trouble with normal': Covid-19's legacy and the multipotentiality for co-creating teaching, learning and assessing

Professor David T Evans, OBE

Although 'The trouble with normal' is a title taken from a queer theory textbook (Warner, 2000), Covid-19 has actually *queered* higher education in ways unimaginable before the pandemic. The pandemic *queers* and challenges many traditional ways we looked at, and provided, teaching, learning and assessing (TLA), especially with specific difficulties faced by health and social care educational providers. Those difficulties have included, but are not limited to, innovative ways of trying to make up for the 'real' human-to-human contact – in class and in professional or clinical practice settings – with a mixed effort and outcome of alternatives. The alternatives have included increased online learning opportunities; more or less blended learning provision; synchronous and asynchronous video and virtual classroom engagement; augmented virtual reality (VR) and artificial intelligence (AI) resources; simulated practice; the gymnastics of flipped classroom pedagogies and techniques (Blázquez et al, 2019), and, of course, the 'workload realism' of the extra hours teachers have put in striving to make all TLA meaningful and rewarding for their students (Arnold, 2021).

Whether we are providers or consumers of TLA, the Covid-19 legacy is making us all scrutinise our provision and expectations of TLA under the microscope. Equally, this microscopic scrutiny of TLA is challenging us to move forward with opportunities, the great potential we learn from this era of current pandemic. There is no going 'back to normal' or back to how things used to be. Why would we? *Why should we?* In fact, as Ashwin (2021) says of students, teachers and institutions, *'the importance [is] of the design of curricula, including assessments, which provide students with access to knowledge which will transform their sense of who they are and what they can do in the world'*. This sentiment is backed up by Sambell and Brown (2021, p 11), when, in relation to changes for assessment strategies, they say: *'one way of supporting this change [...] is to reconceptualise assessment and feedback practices by adopting future-oriented design principles'*.

Students, teachers and our learning institutions now have an unprecedented opportunity to actively participate in the co-creation of our new and evolving 'normal' as a continuous collaborative transformation, inspiring learning partners of today and empowering the academic citizens of tomorrow. Part of this new creation is to see how gains won and developments achieved need to be on-going – future orientated, not going back. Sambell and Brown (2021, p 11) affirm how *we now have a once-in-a-generation opportunity to reimagine assessment for good, rather than simply returning to the status quo'*. For example, a literature review conducted by McDonald et al (2018, p 66) concluded that *'e-based learning and traditional teaching methods used in conjunction with each other create a superior learning style'*. Shaw (2021) adds that an overwhelming percentage of young people going to or currently at university prefer the whole face-to-face on-campus experience, including formal classroom teaching, to counteract what Arnold (2021) refers to as *'the human act of full engagement [which] was undoubtedly compromised'*. So, Covid-19 has made us reconsider our entire approach to TLA. This opportunity helps us to see traditional campus-based and synchronous online 'face-to-face' learning, (often) supplemented with a wide range of asynchronous online provision, not as a case of one thing or the other, an 'either/or' situation, but beneficial for exploring ways to combine the best elements of all across the range of our curricula, to boost the providers' (institutions and teachers) and end-users' (the students or learners) experience.

Developing multipotentialite graduates: motivating passive students into active learners

As with other current-day higher education sector students, health and social care learners have already experienced variable amounts of online teaching and learning provision. This provision, often in contrasting formats, with divergent passive or active learning engagement and variable quality, are an increasing part of undergraduate pre-qualifying curricula. E-learning is also an integral part of post-qualifying continuing personal and professional development too, and through multiple apps (electronic applications or programmes) and devices, operationalised across fields of health and social care professional practice in platforms for learning such as the Social Care Institute for Excellence (SCIE, see www.scie.org.uk/) and e-Learning for Healthcare (e-LfH, see www.e-lfh.org.uk/). In a way, the range of e-TLA can be harnessed and developed to capture best practice and wider potential opportunities for an even greater all-round learning experience, enabling a compassionate 'pedagogy of care' (Arnold, 2021) for a truly responsive community of shared learning values and practice as we move forward from the Covid-19 era.

One dimension of learning frequently left behind, however, is academic assessment (Baughan, 2021). While teachers, institutions and learners have heard calls from many quarters (not least the Covid-19 disruption) to totally redesign their assessment formats and processes – and to *'scale up flexible assessment'* as Sam Elkington (2021, p 38) calls it – higher education institutions often face an additional bind. This bind or responsibility is from practice-based professional, statutory and regulatory bodies who have their own expectations of the hoops they require their registrants to jump through.

Reimagining assessments – a case in point

Many teachers have felt 'thrown in at the deep end' with Covid-19, its numerous lockdowns and rapid shifts to (more or better) online learning opportunities. Individual teachers may be effective educators, facilitating small group tutorials or standing in front of a lecture hall with 200 to 300 students, but how does one manage to be equally as good and effective with e-learning provision and delivery? This does not just mean performing in front of a camera on Zoom or Microsoft Teams, but through a total re-conceptualisation of teaching, learning *and* assessment with formal and specific e-learning pedagogies. In addition, and equally important, is how to manage assessment of learning in new, novel and contemporarily relevant ways (Brown, 2021).

In considering a redesign of assessments, making them genuinely fit for purpose, Dr Joanne Tai (2021) says that teachers and institutions need to be cognisant of our students' diverse and intersecting backgrounds, their learning goals and interests, and their 'futures beyond university'. Such a message is imperative in helping build the multiple forms of potential in our students. To do so effectively, we also need to contemplate the specifics of genuine e-learning pedagogies and andragogies, or what some call *pedandragogies* (Evans, 2020). We cannot simply take our classroom style of teaching and modes of assessment or exam invigilation, and transpose them onto a virtual learning environment (VLE); such a move would be wholly naïve of us, as otherwise expert teachers.

A case in point

One of the exclusively e-learning modules I facilitate is called 'Promoting Sexual Health'. I inherited the assignments: a (sexual) health promotion essay, for Academic Level 6, and a paper-based (sexual) health promotion leaflet, with accompanying theoretical essay, at Level 7. I have now reinvented these assignments, teaching the students how to use and design in Adobe Spark™ and

Adobe PremierRush. At Level 6, the students critically reflect on designing a potential sexual health resource, as an Adobe Spark Page, using all three key functions of Spark (Page, Video and Post/Graphic). At Level 7, they create an actual Adobe Spark (3 elements) resource, ready for disseminating to a client population, and they must also include at least one self-edited video using Adobe PremierRush.

Some technophobic students may be apprehensive, at first, about how they will achieve their learning outcomes. With both early-in-module real-time (online) teaching, supported by asynchronous materials for both the Adobe apps, not only do they all enjoy their subject matter learning and novel assessment [https://spark.adobe.com/page/v3bBVVmXeoeRv/] but they take away with them creative digital skills for the advancement of their professions and a (more) positive attitude to digital literacy (Health Education England, nd).

Digital literacy: Fluency, confidence and competence

Many teachers have struggled with their own, let alone their students', digital upskilling. Over and above the required urgent upskilling, they have had to manage countless 'how to ...' questions about online TLA, particularly in relation to the provision of assessments. Covid-19 assessment policies are not simply about 'no detriment' or being more relaxed about extenuating circumstances applications (Hale, 2021)! No longer in the proverbial sports hall, but now in individual students' own homes, questions have been raised concerning how to invigilate exams, or how to assess physical interactions during virtual OSCEs (objective structured clinical examinations) and equally, how role plays or simulated practice can be facilitated. Quintessentially important, however, is how to ensure equity, quality and inclusivity across mobile devices and internet provision for all students. This last *how to* is especially important when many students may be technologically averse, technophobic, naïve or challenged, or in 'digital poverty' as their home environments or IT resources are poor, as Jisc (2021) calls it. Arnold (2021) states that the pandemic has *'provided HE [higher education] with a grounding reality check on the diversity of student circumstance'*.

On this point of digital poverty, it is equally important to think of the many end users of social work, health and social care, too: the service users, clients or patients. Many service users, even the reluctant ones, may be expected to use IT resources as part of their package of care. They, too, may be digitally naïve or averse, and might need to be taught the skills required for usage, as well as assistance to acquire the necessary physical resources (smartphone, iPad/tablet, etc) especially if on exceptionally low income in the first place. We also need to consider that some students simply do not want to use such electronic resources, and we need to be compassionate in understanding those who are more digitally hesitant or resistant.

Green et al (2019, p 404) say *'effective communication is central to health education and requires consideration of sources, message and audience factors'.* SCIE (2020) poses a crucial question: *'why should social workers [equally, other health and social care professionals, too] develop their digital capabilities?'* A suggested answer, given by SCIE (2020) is to *'promote user and carer involvement'.* Why? Because *'digital technology can enable social workers to enhance the involvement and participation of adults and children in decisions about their care'.* Indeed, the Royal College of Nursing echoed similar sentiments for nurses:

that the organisation should lobby for every nurse to be an e-nurse, able to use data, information, knowledge and technology to maximum effect for patients, carers and service users. These are no longer specialist issues but affect the whole nursing profession, who need to be supported to practise in new and modern ways.

(Royal College of Nursing, 2018, p 4)

Don't just see one! Do one! Teach one!

Other points for consideration include the apparent lack of appropriate pedagogical underpinning for electronic or virtual education, compounded by a lack of practical training skills for teachers and students. This lack of training for teachers goes wider than the skills-based practice of seeing how something is done ('See one'), then practising it ('Do one') and then passing the knowledge on to others ('Teach one'). These learning deficits relate to the philosophical underpinnings of e-TLA through to the simple mechanics of using so many new electronic programmes. This problem is felt no more keenly than in trying to promote a genuine, active-learning, flipped class-room philosophy and associated technique (Blázquez et al, 2019; Evans, 2020). For example, in situations where students 'turn up' for class and expect to be taught something new, expecting them now to actively engage in a pre-session learning experience might be a shock to their system and a challenge for both students and some teachers!

A case in point

A student walked into one of my classes, about an hour late. He was rather irate at missing the first part of the session, but I reassured him that I had pre-made videos on what we were covering, and had already embedded them into his course Moodle site. He then sneered, 'Hu! Whoever looks at Moodle!?' This story highlights some of the struggles in turning around attitudes from spoon-fed, passive learning, often hitherto experienced by many students (and teachers) experiencing the Virtual Learning Environment (VLE) as a repository for documents and reading materials, rather than as a zone for active and proactive engagement.

To turn our VLEs into genuine communities for sharing learning online we need to start by learning how to build on and maximise the platforms we use, especially through adapting and applying relevant aspects of the philosophies of e-pedagogy or e-andragogy, as appropriate, for each different course and set of learners.

A new mindset: A cognitive reorientation of the ways we think of TLA

Included within specific e-pedagogical theories is the need to take an overview, a meta-cognitive approach, to the whole learning process as well as the student's role within it. This metacognitive approach includes answering the 'why' and 'how to' of the very need (the rationale behind) for their cooperation, especially in the more participatory styles required of e-learning engagement. This metacognitive approach to learning also extolls the benefits of active development for the students' own shared learning opportunities, be this in formal sessions or via peer collaboration and support outside formal timetabled learning.

It is important to explain the concept and responsibilities of flipped classroom tech-nique, especially to those who might be wondering why they have been asked to work through resources and materials prior to their shared (virtual or campus) classroom time together (Evans, 2020). In explanation, it is worth clarifying that the modules students undertake, eg for 15 or 30 credits, mean that the all-round learning package should take about 150 to 300 hours, respectively (where one credit equals ten hours of study). Obviously, students do not get all of those hours in classroom, and thus they are already required to do additional self-directed and teacher-driven studies. *That is where 'flipped classroom' technique comes into its own!*

Flipping the classroom learning requires students to work through pre-learning resources, potentially equal to what they would have formerly done in class. These resources might be a week before a timetabled event with the teacher (either on campus or online). In the shared learning time together, rather than the teacher go over the materials from the pre-learning resource again, such as providing a trad-itional lecture, the teacher presumes and expects that the students will have worked through the materials. The teacher and class can then build on this learning, spending time together sharing their outcomes, reflections, ideas, questions and feedback. Such a workshop might also afford time for working in small groups or as a whole class, and to explore further matters to learn even more.

A case in point

When requested to teach on colleagues' programmes the two-hour session I would have formerly presented in a classroom, I now totally re-design in an Adobe Spark Page, such as this one on children, young people and sexual health (Evans, nd). I include elements of text, short videos, links, exercises and feedback, plus some questions to get the students thinking, ready for our time together in a workshop. I then design the workshop – and I call it that, because I expect the students to work at it! – in Mentimeter™.

Using some slides in Mentimeter for my presentation, as I would in PowerPoint™, and others with the various quiz or feedback facility specific to Mentimeter, I can then engage students and require them to contribute in numerous ways. Some engage by turning on their microphone/camera; sometimes in small group activities, or through the anonymity of voting or messaging directly in Menti™ slides. A pdf of the resulting workshop can then be added to the students' VLA, as a backup resource of our shared learning time together.

Tip: If students are quiet or slow to respond, I ask them to consider how it would be in a physical classroom, if they were expected to contribute or respond and there was silence!

By 2021, our TLA really has become technologically dependent, so much so that it is difficult to imagine a class without projector and screens, interactive boards, or Prezi, YouTube, or supported with online engagement. Even using programmes such as Mentimeter in class (whether in a physical room or online) presupposes enough students a) have devices capable of using the programme, and b) know how to use it. The pace at which learning technologies are developing sometimes leaves certain people behind, so, as McDonald et al (2018, p 6) state: *'training and preparation is vital'.*

Empowering carers and enabling clients

It is imperative to consider that empowering social and health care professionals to become more digitally and e-learning experienced needs to have a knock-on effect with clients in their respective fields of practice. It is crucial to take the end-user along with the technological developments, with the aim of such inclusivity not leaving anyone behind. When SCIE (2020) considers the impact on practice, the need is to *'understand the online uses and technology needs of people who use services: [SCIE continues] Social workers should understand how different groups of people with distinct needs, use different online services and technology to support their wellbeing.'* If students and teachers find the pace of e-learning technologies meteoric and possibly difficult, how about clients? How about the populations that might not even be able to afford such technology, let alone have the capability of understanding or using it?

Taking everyone with us

It is crucial we take everyone along with us, so to speak, and leave no one behind as we consider how to capture notions of digital literacy and develop them through fluency and confidence, right through to digital competency. This is as important for the wider academic citizenship achievements of learners as it is for teachers. In fact, various authors of electronic device mediated TLA (e-TLA) are also raising concerns about students who fall behind, simply because they may be too shy or embarrassed about a lack of resources or skills at usage (Jisc, 2021). They may equally be too shy to show their background environments, their home situations. Some might have particular domestic challenges, such as managing or caring for other people and pets at home; schooling children; or trouble with violent or problematic relationships (Burns et al, 2020). Indeed, *fully online courses and blended learning models are being integrated in all manners of instruction at all levels of education to the point that teachers and students alike would have difficulty in participating in many class activities without the Internet'* (Picciano, 2019, p 26). All of these concerns are important to consider, as part of the wider, holistic *persona* of our online teachers and learners and the impact of new realities not just for teaching and learning, but also assessments.

Truly active, participatory and best-practice e-learning provision can be a challenge, of course, for institutional providers (the colleges and universities), the teachers – especially those who often describe themselves as rather camera-shy or technophobic – as well as the student body; with a 'one size doesn't fit all' motif appropriate (Compton and Almpanis, 2018). As teachers providing learning, however, we cannot fail in our quest to deliver the very best opportunities we are able to. Sometimes that means challenging *us* out of our comfort zones, as we embrace and develop these new and future-orientated learning resources.

Future-orientated learning

Particularly for health and social work or care professionals, with their range of clients across all strata of society, across the whole life-course 'from the cradle to the grave', new ways of learning and working will need to be practised and reinforced, not just one-off events, like fads which are easily forgotten. To do so, genuine learning needs to be fourfold, ie to embrace not just the academic *knowledge*, but to enhance positive *attitudes* to new ways of learning, to practise fresh *skills* and reinforce it all with frequent *habits* (described as KASH by Griffith and Burns, 2014).

In light of Covid-19, so many academic quality practices have already been invigorated. These practices include automatic extenuation (extensions) for those students re-deployed to Covid-19 frontline services or vaccination volunteering or equally, 'no detriment' policies for assessment hand-in dates; or judgements on students' diminished capacity for academic achievement. More so, however, there is a need for compassion with frontline students and workers. Higher education institutions must take into consideration the psychological impact the pandemic has had on their learners and staff; the 'above and beyond' work many have done; their grief at (multiple) losses, even the personal suffering of illness and impact of 'long Covid' on themselves or their loved ones.

A leading international expert in assessment development, Professor Sally Brown (see https://sally-brown.net/) also advocates how we need to build in 'compassion', not just across teaching and learning but most especially in our redesign of assessments which are truly responsive to today's professional needs. 'Things can only get better' not by looking back to a fixed point in the past; nor by trying to emulate or re-create that point in time, but by drawing on a plethora of digital resources which support and promote new(er) ways of learning. We also need to enhance the potential from multiple sources of shared learning, and shape this 'new normal' into an active learning (virtual and/or physical) community that is dynamic, compassionate, relevant and inspiring.

What difference can I make?

'Impact' is such a crucial word in today's learning and practice environments. Regarding this chapter, how can social workers, health and other social care professionals use digital technologies to boost their learning potential *and* to make a positive impact on people, systems, services and organisations? SCIE (2020) demonstrates how technology is clearly here to stay, but encourages social and healthcare professionals to do more to take ownership of it, to integrate its use for the greater beneficence of those they care for, and – as demonstrated in the Adobe Spark 'Promoting Sexual Health' assignment described previously – to encourage health and social care professionals to be more proactive in the development and customisation of apps and programmes – to lead, rather than be led, in teaching, learning and assessments.

Three critical questions for practice development, especially in the face of any future lockdowns

The exercise and following questions will enable you to gain maximum benefit from working through this chapter. First, draw up a forcefield analysis (FFA) (Lewin, 1951) to explore the restraining and facilitating forces at play with regards to your own experience of e-TLA at your institution. To do this, in the centre of a blank page write up your aim, ie what you want to achieve in regard to e-TLA. Then explore the hindrances, restraining forces or barriers which can or will block you from achieving your aim. Next, explore the facilitating forces – the enablers – the things that work and will help you achieve your core aim. You may be doing this as a mind-map exercise, and you may be doing it alone or with others. In relation to your FFA, consider the three reflective questions at the end of the chapter.

Summary and conclusion

This chapter has explored numerous dimensions of the Covid-19 legacy on e-teaching, e-learning and e-assessing. It has outlined suggestions for dealing constructively, positively and compassionately with barriers to a whole-system rethink for future directions, inclusive of institutions, teachers and learners. The chapter has also pointed out ways to draw on each other's multiple potential to ensure, future pandemic or not, that there is no going back to an education suited for the past: just forward.

Reflective questions

>> Which and how many of the barriers to you achieving your aim, eg 'to promote (improved) experiences and engagement with electronic device-mediated teaching, learning and assessment (e-TLA)', are within your personal control to overturn or manage more successfully?

>> Who can you recruit to help you minimise the barriers (restraining forces) and maximise the enablers (facilitating forces)?

>> How can you embed your aim, and the positive outcomes, into various e-TLA systems or networks, to ensure they are up and ready, whether or not there are any future disruptions to learning, eg through Covid-19 lockdowns?

This chapter is based on:

Evans, D T (2020) Don't just think outside the box… Exploring e-learning ~ologies in light of Covid-19, an Adobe Spark resource. [online] Available at: https://spark.adobe.com/page/HJXwxytPOXUYH/

and was originally created for my teaching colleagues at the University of Greenwich.

References

Arnold, L (2021) Learning from a Time of Crisis: A Summer Reflection. [online] Available at: https://lydia-arnold.com/2021/08/08/learning-from-a-time-of-crisis-a-summer-reflection/ (accessed 29 December 2021).

Ashwin, P (2021) How Teaching, Learning and Assessment Without Knowledge Undermine the Educational Role of Higher Education. AdvanceHE Assessment Conference 2021. [online] Available at: www.advance-he.ac.uk/programmes-events/events/assessment-and-feedback-symposium-2021 (accessed 29 December 2021).

Baughan, P (ed) (2021) *Assessment and Feedback in a Post-Pandemic Era: A Time for Learning and Inclusion.* AdvanceHE. [online] Available at: www.advance-he.ac.uk/news-and-views/assessment-and-feedback-post-pandemic-era-time-learning-and-inclusion (accessed 29 December 2021).

Blázquez, B O, Masluk, B, Gascon, S, Díaz, R F, Aguilar-Latorre, A, Magallón, I A and Magallón Botaya, R (2019) The Use of Flipped Classroom as an Active Learning Approach Improves Academic Performance in Social Work: A Randomized Trial in a University. *Plos One.* [online] Available at: https://doi.org/10.1371/journal.pone.0214623 (accessed 30 December 2021).

Brown, S (2021) Compassionate Assessment Post-COVID19: Improving Assessment Long Term. QAA Scotland presentation (webcast), Assessment, Learning and Teaching in Higher Education. [online] Available at: https://sally-brown.net/ (accessed 30 December 2021).

Burns, D, Dagnall, N and Holt, M (2020) Assessing the Impact of the COVID-19 Pandemic on Student Wellbeing at Universities in the United Kingdom: A Conceptual Analysis. *Frontiers in Education,* 5: 1–10.

Compton, M and Almpanis, T (2018) One Size Doesn't Fit All: Rethinking Approaches to Continuing Professional Development in Technology Enhanced Learning. *Compass Journal of Learning and Teaching,* 11(1). doi: 10.21100/compass.v11i1.708.

Elkington, S (2021) Scaling Up Flexible Assessment. In Baughan, P (ed) *Assessment and Feedback in a Post-Pandemic Era: A Time for Learning and Inclusion* (pp 31–9). York: AdvanceHE.

Evans, D T (2020) Flipping Classrooms – Guide for Students. [online] Available at: https://youtu.be/5riKyGhw6wA (accessed 20 January 2022).

Evans, D T (nd) Children, Young People and their Sexual Health. [online] Available at: https://express.adobe.com/page/5zN5xpi7dFoF6/ (accessed 20 January 2022).

Green, J, Cross, R, Woodall, J and Tonnes, K (2019) *Health Promotion Planning and Strategies* (4th edition). London: Sage.

Griffith, A and Burns, M (2014) *Teaching Backwards.* Carmarthen: Crown House Publishing Ltd.

Hale, C (2021) *Degree Classification, Grade Inflation and COVID: Lessons from 2019–20.* Higher Education Policy Institute. [online] Available at: www.hepi.ac.uk/2021/04/16/degree-classification-grade-inflation-and-covid-lessons-from-2019-20/ (accessed 11 January 2022).

Health Education England (nd) Digital Literacy of the Wider Workforce. [online] Available at: www.hee.nhs.uk/our-work/digital-literacy (accessed 29 December 2021).

Jisc (2021) Government Action Called for to Lift HE Students out of Digital Poverty. [online] Available at: www.jisc.ac.uk/news/government-action-called-for-to-lift-he-students-out-of-digital-poverty-18-jan-2021 (accessed 29 December 2021).

Lewin, K (1951) *Field Theory in Social Science.* New York: Harper and Row.

McDonald, E W, Boulton, J L and Davis, J L (2018) E-learning and Nursing Assessment Skills and Knowledge: An Integrative Review. *Nurse Education Today*, 66: 166–74. [online] Available at: https://pubmed.ncbi.nlm.nih.gov/29705504/ (accessed 7 February 2022).

Picciano, A G (2019) Blended Learning: Implications for Growth and Access. *Online Learning Journal*: 96–102. [online] Available at: https://olj.onlinelearningconsortium.org/index.php/olj/article/view/1758/590 (accessed 11 January 2022).

Royal College of Nursing (2018) Every Nurse an E-nurse: Insights from a Consultation on the Digital Future of Nursing. [online] Available at: www.rcn.org.uk/professional-development/publications/pdf-007013 (accessed 29 December 2021).

Sambell, K and Brown, S (2021) Changing Assessment for Good: Building on the Emergency Switch to Promote Future-Oriented Assessment and Feedback Designs. In Baughan, P (ed) *Assessment and Feedback in a Post-Pandemic Era: A Time for Learning and Inclusion* (pp 11–21). York: AdvanceHE.

Social Care Institute for Excellence [SCIE] (2020) Digital Capabilities for Social Workers. The Social Care Institute for Excellence. [online] Available at: www.scie.org.uk/social-work/digital-capabilities/capabilities-statement (accessed 11 January 2022).

Shaw, J (2021) *The Vast Majority of Students Want In-Person Learning, Not More Online Classes.* Higher Education Policy Unit. [online] Available at: www.hepi.ac.uk/2021/07/15/the-vast-majority-of-students-want-in-person-learning-not-more-online-classes/ (accessed 11 January 2022).

Tai, J (2021) Assessment for Diversity in the Post-Digital Age. AdvanceHE Assessment Conference 2021. [online] Available at: www.advance-he.ac.uk/programmes-events/events/assessment-and-feedback-symposium-2021 (accessed 11 January 2022).

Warner, M (2000) *The Trouble with Normal: Sex, Politics and the Ethics of Queer Life.* Cambridge, MA: Harvard University Press.

Chapter 2

Reflecting on population health learning in pre-registration paramedic education during a global pandemic

Dr Michael Fanner

Introduction

The pre-hospital emergency care responses in the Covid-19 pandemic would not have been possible without the paramedic profession, mostly working within NHS ambulance services. The pre-registration education that underpins entry to the paramedic profession, therefore, becomes a vital area for considerable reflection on how it prepares paramedics for pandemics and what those involved in paramedic education can learn from this unique period of time. In March 2020, the university sector responses were anticipatory yet fast moving at the start of first implementation of government regulations, aimed at preventing the mass spread of the SARS-CoV-19 virus. Across the sector, difficult decisions were made for the physical closure of university campuses, with rapid transitions to remote and online-only learning, and additionally for health students, postponement or cancellation of clinical placements. Within three months of the University of West London's (UWL) first cohort of the MSc Paramedic Science (Pre-Registration) starting, the pandemic rules were part and parcel of our daily vigilance. Initially, for the UWL student paramedics, their academic experience was not to be so obviously affected as their first term of teaching had been completed and they were to commence their first emergency ambulance placement. However, with the 'touch and go' pace of the significantly increased patient demand (as well as the obvious risk of spread of infection) on NHS ambulance services, clinical placements were postponed, which affected approximately 1000 student paramedics across the year in London alone. This postponement led to a new responsibility on paramedic science academics to provide extra-curricular learning to replace clinical learning through virtual simulation and/or sustain educational enrichment above and beyond 'normal' academic work. The Health and Care Professions Council (HCPC) had advised higher education institutions (HEIs) that approved programmes of study which led to eligibility for a HCPC-registered profession would be able to continue in a flexible manner providing the HCPC standards were maintained.

Ultimately, as educators, we personally knew of the Covid-19-induced occupational stress affecting the ambulance workforce and we continued our concentrated efforts in educating the future paramedics who would almost inevitably become part of the

London Ambulance Service NHS Trust future workforce. So, the decision to postpone the programme would not have benefited anyone in the longer term – neither our students, the ambulance service, the NHS, the patients, nor the public. While the move to remote and online-only learning for most of the first lockdown would be the obvious way forward, students became concerned about a lack of major practical experience in their clinical and theoretical learning for an unknown time period. This practical experience would ultimately consolidate their proficiencies to qualify and register as a paramedic. Managing this student concern was unique to non-clinical programmes of study, so ensuring and maximising the 'virtual' student experience became challenging for academics and students alike due to the 'uncharted waters' that the pandemic had brought.

Organisation of the chapter

First, this chapter will provide a brief history of the evolution and professionalisation of paramedic education, from practical training through to the development of higher education programmes, in the advancement of enhancing pre-hospital care to patients, illuminating the greater need for the public health curriculum and utilisation of student paramedics in pandemic responses. Secondly, an exploration takes place into how the public health curriculum can be designed in pre-registration paramedic education in both non-pandemic and pandemic times. Lastly, this chapter brings together the recent literature on the Covid-19 pandemic response experiences of student paramedics across the globe.

A brief history of paramedic education

Historically, the evolution and professionalisation of ambulance workforce education has significantly transformed from the 'stretcher-bearer' requirements (Williams et al, 2009; First et al, 2012) or offering a 'deliver first aid and transport model' (O'Meara, 2009) to a regulated healthcare profession, namely a paramedic able to problem solve and provide solutions within time-pressured, pre-hospital environments (O'Meara, 2009). Within this professionalisation, pre-registration paramedic education has rapidly advanced from the first 'in-house' ambulance service paramedic training scheme in Brighton in the 1970s (Van de Gaag and Donaghy, 2013) to a predominantly higher education model with mandated clinical placements in approved practice learning partners (eg NHS ambulance services) across the UK. This growth of professionalisation and scope of practice in pre-registration paramedic education means that patients ultimately receive better care and can (although not exclusively) be treated at home without the need to go to hospital (Bigham et al, 2013). Eaton (2019, p 1) rightly observes that *'not all paramedics wear green'* and this is, by and large, because their pre-registration education offers great transferability of knowledge, skills, capabilities and values to other clinical settings, such as emergency departments (eg Clarke, 2019), hospices (eg Singer, 2021) and primary and urgent care (eg Eaton et al, 2020). While these non-traditional settings can be considered as appropriate diversification of the paramedic profession, public perceptions may not recognise these professional movements.

In the UK, paramedics have required state registration since 2000 and are regulated by the HCPC, who also set, maintain, and monitor pre-registration education standards. Certainly, since the introduction of state regulation and registration, the profession has placed greater emphasis on an ambitious model of paramedicine beyond the 'scoop and run' or 'only convey to hospital' approach, which is still a perception of paramedicine for a majority of the public. This ambitious model characteristically aims to distinguish a unique contribution within the multi-disciplinary team, ie autonomous out-of-hospital or pre-hospital clinical decision-making and intervention(s) (Donaghy, 2008; McCann et al, 2013) and experts in episodic biopsychosocial care, a unique feature that I would also add. This professional aspiration is congruent with Lord Carter's review into unwarranted variation in NHS Ambulance Trusts (NHS England, 2018), who identified that the NHS could save £500 million if more patients were better assessed during the 999 call and/or treated in the pre-hospital environment by paramedics, avoiding the need for an unnecessary conveyance to hospital. Lord Carter's review challenges the traditional pattern of ambulance practice (attendance, stabilisation and conveyance) sustainability in use of resources for patients who are now older, sicker and have more complex exacerbations of long-term conditions, when more complex decision-making and discharge or referral plans are now required. The review's findings support the need for paramedic education to go way beyond the historic, biomedically-centric episodic care delivered and to take into account models of health at population levels such as public health, which is observed in the College of Paramedics (CoP) (2019) curriculum guidance (the UK's professional body for paramedics).

The CoP (2019) curriculum guidance aimed at HEIs specifies greater granularity in comparison to the HCPC (2014) Standards of Proficiency (SoPs) for paramedics (and certainly the right way around!). While the CoP curriculum guidance is not mandatory, in order to become a HCPC-approved programme, it offers educational aspiration to the future workforce as well as influencing the content of future HCPC SoPs. Now in its fifth iteration, the curriculum guidance demonstrates the breadth of learning that UK student paramedics undertake. I have highlighted key areas of the guidance that have direct relevance to Covid-19 at a population health level, which are:

» public health;

» health promotion;

» resilience and disaster preparedness;

» health psychology;

» sociology of health.

O'Meara et al (2017) have observed that paramedic education places great centricity on emergency medicine curricula (understandably), and this, along with 'packed' programme planners, reduces the possibility (or creativity) for programmes to include more public health content. However, O'Meara et al also note that paramedic higher education programmes can be flexible in how they are organised, so increasing public health content is entirely possible. A reason for this limitation may be that the paramedic science academic discipline requires more explicit inter-disciplinary input from other academic disciplines such as specialist community public health nursing, public health medicine, community development and epidemiology.

For context-sake, despite this advancement in pre-registration paramedic education and diversification of settings, there has been accelerated and paradoxical introduction of differing strata of very basically skilled ambulance staff (for example, emergency care assistants), most often driven by employer and service provision needs, as Whitmore and Furber (2006) point out. Ambulance personnel with basic skills have always been in existence (with varying role titles) but are limited in what they can offer professionally to patients in the pre-hospital environment when compared with paramedics. The professional differences in the patient offer potentially become problematic as all ambulance staff wear green uniforms. When concentrating on the sole visibility (and value) of paramedics in ambulance services, two situations potentially occur: 1) paramedics become diluted in workforce numbers, and 2) all staff are perceived as 'paramedics' from a layperson's perspective (regardless of rank, role bars and epaulettes). A recent UK Secretary of State for Health and Member of Parliament publicly called paramedics 'ambulance drivers'. Many, if not all, NHS ambulance services having rolling vacancy advertisements for paramedics and there is a clear demand for more people to enter the paramedic profession.

Anecdotally, the majority of the public expect the ambulance service to be quick and responsive to assess and treat their emergency and urgent care needs (in a suspected or expected paramedic capacity) and convey to hospital, and it is unlikely the pandemic changed this perception, other than to increase frustration in delay in response or in receiving a different response to what they may have anticipated. So, the paramedic profession potentially begins to fall into a mixed yet highly charged political and public portrayal of two extremes (or somewhere in between): 'ambulance drivers who basically should treat and convey to hospital when called upon' versus 'evidence-based pre-hospital care professionals who can make safe, complex and ethical decisions, with sometimes non-conveyance outcomes over the phone or in person'. Similar political and public discourse problems can be seen in parallel within nursing workforce discourse (eg Rafferty, 2018). It is the latter portrayal that the profession must continue to advocate beyond paramedics through research inquiry, public education and political lobbying. Lay perceptions of pre-registration paramedic education developments may be very limited, leading to a potential hinderance to the forward momentum and public support for advancing professional education in paramedicine, including using student paramedics as part of pandemic responses, increasing non-repayable funding available for studying paramedic science, and perhaps also part-time self-funded study options.

This section has essentially outlined that pre-registration paramedic education has always been embedded in clinical practice but is now structured through formalised learning (Laurillard, 2012) in a higher education model, together with *probably* as much, if not more 'clinical' training (whether actual or simulated) in current paramedic education programmes than historical, shorter, in-house paramedic courses. In a recent academic commentary, Whitfield et al (2020) argue that student paramedics may have been under-utilised in the Covid-19 pandemic even though their education is premised on their development to become *'safe, adaptable and ethical clinicians who can analyse situations and react appropriately in a dynamic and continually challenging environment'* (Whitfield et al, 2020, p 2). Whitfield et al also highlight that when compared to other types of pandemic responders such as health volunteers with basic training, student paramedics are far more versatile and useful in times of national emergency need.

Identifying the public health curriculum in paramedic education design

Building upon the CoP (2019) curriculum guidance and O'Meara et al's (2017) findings from the literature, the UWL MSc Paramedic Science programme offers a first-year 30 credit module entitled *Population Health and Behavioural Science for Paramedic Practice*. The module introduces the principles of population dynamics and healthcare demand, in order to help paramedic science students understand how service constraints impact on population need and dispatch decision-making in ambulance practice. The module provides teaching and learning on recognising the impact of the psychosocial and economic determinants of health on populations and individuals and contributes to improvement in health outcomes through multi-agency working and the use of behavioural interventions in patient contacts. This includes developing an understanding of the health system interfaces which impact on ambulance service response and deployment. From a UK Quality Code for Higher Education (QAA, 2014) perspective, this module requires learners to demonstrate a systematic, extensive and comparative understanding of the key population health topics within the current multi-disciplinary knowledge base(s), while also (critically) appraising and appreciating ambiguity, uncertainty and the limitations of population health knowledge in a systematic and wide-ranging way, when applied to paramedic science. A small number of taught session examples of the module can be found in Table 2.1.

Table 2.1 Selected examples of taught sessions on the population health and behavioural science module

Introduction to Public Health: UK and Global Challenges
Topics included:
• identifying local, national and international public health priorities;
• principles of health protection and promotion at individual and population levels in national and international contexts, eg antimicrobial stewardship, cold weather plan, heatwave plan and pandemic influenza plan.
Appraising Demographic and Epidemiological Data for Paramedic Practice
Topics included:
• demographic and epidemiological data interpretation for paramedic practice;
• case definition and different data used in determining medical diagnosis;
• principles of screening versus testing;
• epidemiological monitoring.
Sociological Considerations to Health and Illness
Topics included:
• applied sociology of health and illness in paramedic practice;
• political ideologies in state health provision;
• the construction of social problems;
• theoretical consideration for the biomedical model underpinning JRCALC assessments and interventions;
• critically appraising 'person-centred', 'lived experience' and 'biopsychosocial' concepts in paramedic practice.

Population Health Needs and Ambulance Deployment

Topics included:

- resource utilisation and organisation in ambulance services to meet population health needs (including multi-agency working);
- signposting/referral systems eg ambulance response and deployment decisions;
- local strategic health needs assessments;
- inequality and healthcare resource use in different social groups.

At the start of the pandemic and its unfolding, there was a new pressure on academics to ensure that students could begin to make sense of the daily (or at least weekly) media-facilitated, public display of conflict and clashing between ardent advocates of evidence-based medicine, policy advisors, clinicians and politicians on government pandemic decisions (Watson and McCrae, 2020). This public conflict and clashing, which led to a confusing public discourse, was often a result of the different interpretation of the same (emerging) evidence on infectivity and transmissibility of the SARS-CoV-19 virus with the introduction of wide-ranging preventative measures such as handwashing, face masks, social distancing and the implementation of lockdowns, and latterly vaccines (Fanner and Maxwell, 2021). The UWL MSc Paramedic Science academic team created a 'wholesale' response to framing the emerging Covid-19 condition and pandemic across modular learning where appropriate.

Table 2.1 illustrates a sample of what the UWL student paramedics learnt in the three months running up to the implementation of pandemic rules, meaning they were able to start 'dissecting' the pandemic decision-making and make sense of the pandemic through a (broader and post-graduate) paramedicine lens. While the module teaching had finished by the time the pandemic rules came into place, the module continued regular virtual learning contact, facilitating either taught sessions or academic journal clubs on topics that arose in the government briefings (eg herd immunity, the emerging case definition of Covid-19 and social distancing measures). As the module leader and lecturer, I had to rapidly interpret the daily changes in government public health measures through an academic and professional lens based on my own professional learning as a specialist community public health nurse and post-doctoral research literacy. Sometimes I felt self-doubt as a result of the differences between my academic and professional opinion and the UK government pandemic decisions. For example, the taught session I designed on the theoretical basis of 'herd immunity' was potentially contradictory at the time as it was not 'in line' with the UK government's pandemic ideology of 'following the science'. We have since learnt, through public inquiry, that the conscious emphasis of immunity through natural infection spread approach taken by the UK government was disastrous, leading to thousands of unnecessary Covid-19 deaths.

The online journal clubs were effective when learning design explicated the online teaching and learning experience (eg based on Laurillard's (2002) conversational framework), as well as explicit learning types such as Laurillard's (2012) six learning types (acquisition, inquiry, discussion, practice, production, collaboration). Two papers used in the journal clubs covered the original retrospective cohort study on the clinical course and risk factors for mortality of adult inpatients with Covid-19 in Wuhan (Zhou et al, 2020) and an earlier 2004 comparative study on the public's response to Severe Acute Respiratory Syndrome (SARS) in Toronto and the United States (Blendon et al, 2004). The journal clubs worked incredibly well at reflecting both forwards and backwards, and gave students stability in their daily lives as learners as well as citizens.

Concentrating educational efforts on the pandemic experience of teaching and learning through explicit learning types, as previously discussed, may point towards a solution of the existing research findings on online or hybrid learning experiences of student paramedics during the Covid-19 pandemic. The research findings within the literature highlight the need to create more social connection opportunities with campus closure (Whitfield et al, 2021), supporting the development of positive coping strategies (Williams et al, 2021) and increasing the motivation to learn online when face-to-face teaching is favoured (Allfred et al, 2021).

The student paramedic experience of the Covid-19 pandemic

On 3 April 2020, a joint statement by the HCPC, the Chief Allied Health Professions Officers of the four nations of the UK and the Council of Deans of Health was published that outlined how allied health professions students (including paramedics) would be supported to respond to the Covid-19 pandemic. The joint statement (HCPC et al, 2020) quickly established that any intervention they would put into place would need to balance the needs of patients, frontline health professionals and students, to enable students to offer their support to the NHS with the least disruption to their education. The joint statement made four over-arching points:

1. Automatic (temporary) registration for final year students who had completed their clinical placements with approval from their HEI to enable them to work at NHS Agenda for Change (AfC) Band 5 pay. Full registration

would occur later, as per normal processes, in some cases with additional theoretical learning and assessment.

2. Final year students who had not completed their clinical placements, second year of their BSc (third year in Scotland) or first year of an MSc could support the NHS in a paid support worker role, renumerated at NHS AfC Band 3, and the hours undertaken would go towards their required practice hours (determined by each HEI). This second point recognised progressive and sustained clinical learning while bearing in mind reduced placement capacity in the health system.

3. All other students would continue their university programmes but have placements paused. This third point meant that students were to focus on the theoretical parts of their education (with HEIs encouraged to bring academic learning forward), with clinical learning requirements to be achieved later in their programme.

4. All students were able to volunteer to support the front line in their spare time, which would make no contribution to their clinical learning hours.

It should be noted that students who fell under point two may have been deployed anywhere in roles that may or may not have been directly relevant to their usual clinical environments, such as a hospital ward rather than an ambulance. Naturally, many student paramedics sought to volunteer their support to local ambulance services – even offering to just restock and prepare ambulances for frontline work.

Following the onset of the pandemic, UK ambulance services were faced with four main challenges, which Emmerson (2021) observed as:

1. difficulties in answering and clinically triaging unprecedented increased numbers of 999 and 111 calls (in March 2020, 999 calls doubled, and 111 calls trebled);

2. being able to find enough additional vehicles;

3. being able to find enough clinical and operational staff from answering calls to clinical response to logistics to vehicle maintenance;

4. the loss of up to 20 per cent of workforce to Covid-related sickness and self-isolation.

In order to deal with these difficulties, ambulance services thought creatively about how this increased demand for services could be met, which included rapidly recruiting from a wide range of public sector workers (such as firefighters, the military), voluntary workers (eg community first responders) and student paramedics to work on the front line (Corr, 2020) or using first and second year student paramedics to work in 999 call centres (see Emmerson, 2021). St John Ambulance (NHS England's resilience ambulance service) created opportunities for second- and third-year student paramedics to have their prior learning recognised to operate at emergency ambulance crew level in assisting frontline calls. So, it is evident that student paramedics played a part in helping the ambulance services but there is currently no formal data that captures their full and collective contribution.

There is some published literature (primary research and academic commentary) that identifies the student paramedic experience of the Covid-19 pandemic from Australia (Whitfield et al, 2020; Perkins et al, 2020; Williams et al, 2021; Whitfield et al, 2021), England (Miller, 2021), Norway (Häikiö et al, 2021) and the United States (Allfred et al, 2021). A number of key considerations on how student paramedics can contribute frontline services during a health crisis or pandemic can be identified from the primary research findings as follows.

Miller (2021) undertook a small qualitative study exploring a new, paid, hybrid role for student paramedics working as one half of a double-crewed ambulance to increase workforce capacity in the East of England NHS ambulance service during the first wave. Miller found that there was broad positivity about this role with perceptions that this type of role could continue post-pandemic, but also identified that issues regarding job descriptions and working conditions were not always clear-cut and many felt they should have been given driver training.

Williams et al (2021) identified from the qualitative interviews in their mixed methods study that almost all of the 17 undergraduate paramedicine students reported that they were not dissuaded from studying to be a paramedic since the outbreak and were aware of the 'dangers' that may face them on qualification. Only two of the 17 participants were concerned about undertaking placements during the pandemic, but this was in light of the fear of contracting and passing the infection on to others. The other participants perceived themselves to be fit and healthy and if they were to contract Covid-19, they would be 'fine'.

Häikiö et al (2021) identified that 36.7 per cent (n = 40/109) of study participants (student paramedics) undertook patient-related healthcare work during the pandemic, with 20 in study-related clinical placement in the ambulance service. A further 10 per cent (n = 11/109) undertook vehicle decontamination and logistical work in the ambulance service. Häikiö et al found that student paramedics were motivated to participate in the pandemic response, despite poor personal protective equipment supplies. Häikiö et al asserted that student paramedics should be considered as a valuable operational resource during crisis, and student paramedics with *'theoretical knowledge and simulation-acquired skills in emergency medicine, trauma and disaster management and with clinical experience should be considered for unsupervised clinical work as part of a national response to a pandemic or other major disasters'* (2021, p 11).

From reviewing this small amount of literature, there is an apparent appetite from student paramedics and their educators to consider students in the pandemic response(s) with their pre-hospital focused acquired knowledge, skills, capabilities and values. Safeguards for student participation do, of course, need to be considered in respect to patient safety and practice supervision requirements, together with professional indemnity and insurance cover.

Conclusion

In summary, student paramedics bring a unique contribution to the table that differs from other healthcare students and are potentially more likely to 'deal with' Covid-19 positive patients effectively because they:

» want to be considered on par with other students and be made useful to health and care systems with their developing paramedic knowledge, skills, values and behaviours, thereby encouraging their life-long ambition and drive to want to help;

» focus on episodic biopsychosocial care in the main, providing a triaging mindset in symptom-led assessment and intervention with greater confidence in managing uncertainty;

» have significant experience in responding to unplanned and emergency care needs of patients, including enhanced communication and history-taking skills;

» have competence in assessing and treating patients in time-pressurised environments, utilising both lifesaving (for example, ABCDE) and systems-based (eg organ-focused) assessment models, without great reliance upon definitively diagnoseable conditions with familiar assessment and intervention trajectories;

» have competence in immediate and advanced life support, such as resuscitation and managing critically unwell patients;

» have critical awareness of human factors when dealing with emergencies;

» have a specific curriculum focused on public health that will inevitably grow.

This list is purposively simplistic and aspirational and it would not be appropriate to deploy all student paramedics, for example first year students, or those who are subject to action plans. This chapter has also considered how explicit reflection on the academic performance level of a paramedic programme (eg master's level) as well as explicit learning design can help support and promote student learning experience during a health crisis or pandemic and post-pandemic. This chapter continues the long-standing academic discourse that demonstrates how university education (in this case, at master's level) can truly benefit the paramedic profession, especially in the profession's contribution to national health emergencies and at the same time developing a clinically and academically resilient future workforce able to comprehend new and emerging diseases (such as Covid-19) and new or resultant clinical practices.

Reflective questions

» Since the pandemic, how might the public's perceptions change with what they expect from the education of health and social care professions?

» In what ways did university or practice educators adapt the health and social care professional curriculum in the Covid-19 pandemic (or could adapt in a future pandemic) that would enhance personal and academic resilience in students?

» How might university or practice educators consider using online teaching and learning differently moving forward?

Acknowledgements

This chapter is dedicated to the first UWL student paramedics – Antonia, Becky, Derry, Ellie, Georgie, Katherine, Kez, Jack, Rob and Will – for their utmost professionalism and ownership in striving for the best possible learning experience throughout the first and second waves of the Covid-19 pandemic (the time I spent with them). I would also like to express my gratitude to the London Ambulance Service NHS Trust for developing opportunities for student paramedics to work within their 111 service, as this opportunity served as great insight for the UWL students. I would also like to acknowledge Neil Larman, Professional Lead for Paramedics at UWL, for his intelligence, wisdom, support and leadership during my lecturing practice on the MSc.

References

Allred, S, McCarthy, K and Fisher, J (2021) The COVID-19 Pandemic's Impact on Students in a Paramedic Study Program. *Journal of Security, Intelligence and Resilience Education*, 11(1): 1–24.

Bigham, B L, Kennedy, S M, Drennan, I and Morrison, L J (2013) Expanding Paramedic Scope of Practice in the Community: A Systematic Review of the Literature. *Prehospital Emergency Care*, (17): 361–72.

Blendon, R J, Benson, J M, Des Roches, C M, Raleigh, E and Taylor-Clark, K (2004) The Public's Response to Severe Acute Respiratory Syndrome in Toronto and the United States. *Clinical Infectious Diseases*, 38: 925–31.

Clarke, A (2019) What are the Clinical Practice Experiences of Specialist and Advanced Paramedics Working in Emergency Department Roles? A Qualitative Study. *British Paramedic Journal*, 4(3): 1–7.

College of Paramedics (2019) *Paramedic Curriculum Guidance* (5th edition). College of Paramedics.

Corr, S (2020) East of England Ambulance Service Appeals for Volunteers to Help Cope with Coronavirus Crisis. *Bishop's Stortford Independent*. [online] Available at: www.bishopsstortfordindependent.co.uk/news/ambulance-service-for-herts-and-essex-needs-1-000-temps-and-volunteers-9105692/ (accessed 29 July 2021).

Donaghy, J (2008) Higher Education for Paramedics – Why? *Journal of Paramedic Practice*, 1(1): 31–5.

Eaton, G (2019) Paramedic. *noun. British Paramedic Journal*, 4(2): 1–3.

Eaton, G, Wong, G, Williams, V, Roberts, N and Mahtani, K R (2020) Contribution of Paramedics in Primary and Urgent Care: A Systematic Review. *British Journal of General Practice*, 70(695): e421–e426.

Emmerson, G (2021) In Every Crisis, There Is Also Opportunity. National Leadership Centre. [online] Available at: www.nationalleadership.gov.uk/public-leaders-report-2021/supporting-the-nhs-in-its-hour-of-need/london-ambulance-service/ (accessed 11 January 2022).

Fanner, M and Maxwell, E (2021) Children with Long Covid: Co-producing a Specialist Community Public Health Nursing Response. *Journal of Health Visiting*, 9(10): 418–24.

First, S, Tomlins, L and Swinburn, A (2012) From Trade to Profession: The Professionalisation of the Paramedic Workforce. *Journal of Paramedic Practice*, 4(7): 378–81.

Häikiö, K, Andersen, J V, Bakkerud, M, Christiansen, C R, Rand, K and Staff, T (2021) A Retrospective Survey Study of Paramedic Students' Exposure to SARS-CoV-2, Participation in the COVID-19 Pandemic Response and Health-Related Quality of Life. *Scandinavian Journal of Trauma, Resuscitation and Emergency Medicine*, 29: 153.

Health and Care Professions Council (HCPC) (2014) Standards of Proficiency for Paramedics. Health and Care Professions Council.

Health and Care Professions Council, NHS England and NHS Improvement and Health Education England, Llywodraeth Cymru Welsh Government, Department of Health (Northern Ireland), Scottish Government and Council of Deans of Health (2020) Joint statement on how we will support and enable the student allied health professional workforce to respond to the Covid-19 outbreak. [online] Available at: www.councilofdeans.org.uk/wp-content/uploads/2020/04/Joint-statement-on-how-we-will-support-and-enable-the-student-allied-health-professional-workforce-to-respond-to-the-Covid-19-V3.pdf (accessed 2 January 2022).

Laurillard, D (2002) *Rethinking University Teaching. A Conversational Framework for the Effective Use of Learning Technologies*. London: Routledge.

Laurillard, D (2012) *Teaching as a Design Science: Building Pedagogical Patterns for Learning and Technology*. London: Routledge.

McCann, L, Granter, E, Hyde, P and Hassard, J (2013) Still Blue-Collar After all These Years? An Ethnography of the Professionalisation of Emergency Ambulance Work. *Journal of Management Studies*, 50: 5.

Miller, J (2021) PP26: Stepping Up: Interviews with Student Paramedics and Lecturers about a Scheme to Increase Workforce Capacity Within an English Ambulance Service During the First Wave of the COVID-19 Pandemic. Poster Presentation. *Emergency Medicine Journal*, 38: 9.

NHS England (2018) *Operational Productivity and Performance in English NHS Ambulance Trusts.* [online] Available at: www.england.nhs.uk/wp-content/uploads/2019/09/Operational_productivity_and_performance_NHS_Ambulance_Trusts_final.pdf (accessed 2 January 2022).

O'Meara, P F (2009) Paramedics Marching Toward Professionalism. *Australasian Journal of Paramedicine,* 7: 1.

O'Meara, P F, Furness, S and Gleeson, R (2017) Educating Paramedics for the Future: A Holistic Approach. *Journal of Health and Human Services Administration,* 40(2): 219–53.

Perkins, A, Kelly, S, Dumbleton, H and Whitfield, S (2020) Pandemic Pupils: COVID-19 and the Impact on Student Paramedics. *Australasian Journal of Paramedicine,* 17: 1–4.

Quality Assurance Agency for Higher Education (QAA) (2014) *UK Quality Code for Higher Education. Part A: Setting and Maintaining Academic Standards. The Frameworks for Higher Education Qualifications of UK Degree-Awarding Bodies.* Quality Assurance Agency for Higher Education.

Rafferty, A M (2018) Nurses as Change Agents for a Better Future in Health Care: The Politics of Drift and Dilution. *Health Economics, Policy and Law,* 13: 475–91.

Singer, M (2021) P-123 The Role of a Paramedic in a Community Hospice/Palliative/End-of-life Care Team. *BMJ Supportive and Palliative Care,* 11(2): A53.

Van der Gaag, A and Donaghy, J (2013) Paramedics and Professionalism: Looking Back and Looking Forwards. *Journal of Paramedic Practice,* 5(1): 8–10.

Watson, R and McCrae, N (2020) Will Evidence-Based Medicine be Another Casualty of COVID-19? *Journal of Advanced Nursing,* 76(12): 3228–30.

Whitfield, S, MacQuarrie, A and Boyle, M (2020) Trained, Ready but Under-Utilised: Using Student Paramedics During a Pandemic. *Australasian Journal of Paramedicine,* 17: 1–3.

Whitfield, S, Perkins, A, Kelly, S and Dumbleton, H (2021) Uncharted Waters: The Effects of COVID-19 on Student Paramedics. *Australasian Journal of Paramedicine,* 18: 1–7.

Whitmore, D and Furber, R (2006) The Need for a Professional Body for UK Paramedics. *Australasian Journal of Paramedicine,* 4: 1.

Williams, B, Onsman, A and Brown, T (2009) From Stretcher-Bearer to Paramedic: The Australian Paramedics' Move Towards Professionalisation. *Australasian Journal of Paramedicine,* 7(4): 1–12.

Williams, B, King, C, Shannon, B and Gosling, C (2021) Impact of COVID-19 on Paramedicine Students: A Mixed Methods Study. International Emergency Nursing, 56: 100996.

Zhou, F, Yu, T, Du, R, Fan, G, Liu, Y, Liu, Z, Xiang, J, Wang, Y, Song, B, Gu, X, Guan, L, Wei, Y, Li, H, Wu, X, Xu, J, Tu, S, Zhang, Y, Chen, H and Cao, B (2020) Clinical Course and Risk Factors for Mortality of Adult Inpatients with COVID-19 in Wuhan, China: A Retrospective Cohort Study. *The Lancet,* 395: 1054–62.

Chapter 3

How Covid-19 has impacted upon the practice learning experience of pre-registration nursing students

Barbara Hoyle

Introduction

In March 2020 all UK universities instigated 'lockdown' and closed their doors to students and academic staff in a government response to slowing the spread of Covid-19. Six months previously, a number of universities also began implementing the *Future Nurse: Standards of proficiency for registered nurses* (Nursing and Midwifery Council [NMC], 2018a) following an intensive NMC approval process. The process is based on the submission of evidence to ascertain whether universities and their practice learning partners can meet the requirements of the NMC education and training standards as well as the relevant programme standards as determined in each 'gateway':

» gateway 1 – standards framework for nursing and midwifery education;

» gateway 2 – standards for student supervision and assessment;

» gateway 3 – programme standards;

» approval visit from NMC representatives.

The new standards were heralded as offering a more flexible approach to pre-registration nurse education and, in particular, to practice-based learning which was largely reflected in the overhaul of the practice assessment process. However, there was also the inclusion of more advanced clinical 'proficiencies' to be achieved by all newly qualified nursing registrants as outlined in Annexe B: Nursing procedures of the *Future Nurse* standards (NMC, 2018a).

This chapter attempts to capture the lived experience of the Covid-19 pandemic on managing the practice learning experience of pre-registration nursing students from the perspective of a Head of Practice Education with a particular focus on the unprecedented challenges of transitioning onto a new curriculum during this period, and the necessity of an accelerated technical shift in communication and learning approaches.

Transition

Transitioning to the new NMC (2018a) standards required a university managed programme of preparation for both academic and practice staff in order to meet the requirements of an NMC validation. There were two key differences to that of the previous NMC (2008) education and training standards. The practice assessment had changed significantly – 'essential skills' had been replaced with the more clinically advanced 'proficiencies'. Gone were the roles of mentor, sign off mentor and accompanying annual updates and mentor registers, to be replaced instead with practice assessors – practice supervisors who, although they had attended preparatory workshops, were no longer required to achieve an equivalent of a university validated mentor module. Nurse lecturers now assumed a new role of academic assessors who for the first time were charged to liaise with practice assessors to confirm student progression in practice as well as academically.

Despite reverting from the previous process driven standards (NMC, 2008) to implementing an outcome focussed model, the NMC were uncharacteristically specific in defining the new assessor and supervisor roles in *Realising Professionalism. Standards for Education and Training. Part 2: Standards for Student Supervision and Assessment* (NMC, 2018b). This specificity has relevance when in other respects the NMC offered only minimal guidance to managing the logistics of achieving practice assessments and quality assurance processes. Even without the additional considerations brought on by the pandemic, it was becoming increasingly apparent that for students in all four fields of nursing to be enabled to achieve all Annexe B proficiencies in clinical practice was, in many instances, going to be a challenge.

The practice learning experience in 'lockdown'

On 25 March 2020, the NMC published their response to the Covid-19 emergency (NMC, 2020a) and instigated the *Emergency Standards for Nursing and Midwifery Education* (NMC, 2020b). As the global pandemic had taken hold throughout the UK, the emergency standards became the initial road map to keep the practice education wheels moving. However, the challenges of managing swift and sweeping changes were unprecedented and were to significantly impact upon students, lecturers and practice staff alike.

The emergency standards considered each student nurse year group, taking into account their practice supervision requirements and clinical safety factors. All first-year students were withdrawn from clinical placements to continue their programme in theoretical studies only. It was envisaged that the requisite practice hours would be achieved later in their programme. However, as it later transpired, this was to become a major challenge the following year. Second year students and those in the first six months of their third year could choose to 'opt in' to an extended paid placement for 80 per cent of the time with the remaining 20 per cent spent in theoretical learning if they met specific criteria. Likewise, students in the final six months of their programme could 'opt-in' to a 100 per cent extended paid placement endorsed with protected learning time. The differences between each year group, especially those cohorts who started their programme of study outside of the traditional academic year, meant the potential for greater confusion.

Many universities adopted the approach that was pragmatic but also ensured the occupational health and safety of students. Students who might otherwise have been eligible for a paid placement were exempt if:

» they were known to require additional support and supervision in practice or were on an existing action plan;

» they were 'shielding' a member of their family;

» they were medically vulnerable as identified through an occupational health Covid-19 assessment.

So, apart from first year students, there were also significant numbers of second and third year nursing students relying on online learning to enable them to continue with their studies.

Digital movement in university education

The haste with which virtual classrooms were created and the mass introduction of virtual lectures was unparalleled in the long-standing tradition of careful implementation of new teaching, learning and assessment strategies within universities. While online learning had been an evolving technology for at least 20 years (Taft et al, 2011) it is not a simple transformative process to apply to nurse education, principally because it must take into account both the theoretical and practice requirements situated within a professional regulatory standards framework (Smith et al, 2009). As lecturers were quickly acclimatising to the new technologies and revising all their teaching materials into a digital format, so too were the students adapting to a cultural shift to their previous experience of face-to-face learning.

Systematic appraisal of the nursing educational research to date has identified the benefits of online learning and cites its flexibility and ability to promote deeper learning (Webb et al, 2017). Such evidence offered a degree of assurance that students were not necessarily going to be disadvantaged by transferring over to a wholesale package of online learning. Perhaps the positive spin to lockdown was that it offered students the opportunity to plan their own learning and revision at times convenient to them. Online learning materials could be accessed from any location at any time and as many times as required (Barker et al, 2013) and were therefore instrumental in encouraging the notion of self-directed lifelong learning and ensuring current and evidence-based practice as sanctioned within the code (NMC, 2018c), a notion also expected of, or at least encouraged in, students in the clinical learning environment.

Further benefits of becoming familiar with digital technology are cited as the pre-paratory experience students acquire for twenty-first-century clinical practice as highlighted in both the NMC (2018a) *Future Nurse* standards and the *NHS Long Term Plan* (NHS, 2019). As one of its aims, the plan sets out the proposal to provide main-stream digitally-enabled primary and outpatient care and goes further in section 5.1 to describe the NHS as a *'hotbed of innovation and technological revolution in practice'*. Doubtless, the pandemic has accelerated the arrival of mainstream digital medicine, but conversely this has also had an unforeseen outcome in relation to the student experience of clinical practice and indirectly on placement capacity.

Anecdotally, it became clear not all students enjoy online learning. The perception, too, that all students are computer literate is erroneous, particularly among the more mature students (Bramer, 2020). Likewise, not all students have home computers and in the absence of being able to access library computers they reported the necessity of relying on friends and families for use of their computers to write theory assignments and then using their own smartphones to join virtual classrooms and webinars. Equally, problems with poor internet connectivity created barriers to learning and the neces-sity of social isolation negated the benefits of face-to-face classroom discussions and student–lecturer interactions, although conversely, this was mitigated to some degree by the virtual classroom (Bramer, 2020). However, universities became increasingly concerned about the deterioration in the mental well-being of their students and we are only beginning to understand how long-term social isolation can have a detri-mental effect on mental health.

Of paramount importance from the outset was the provision of pastoral support to all students, particularly those who were in practice – a fact recognised by the universities and underlined by Health Education England (HEE) (2020a) in their publication *Student Support Guidance During COVID-19 Outbreak*. Regular digital meetings between course leaders with each cohort became the norm and also between personal tutors and their students, as reported in frequent regional HEE meetings. HEE also used webinars and online meetings to share current information with students and provide a platform for reciprocal discussions and sharing of concerns (O'Gorman et al, 2020). However, by November 2020 the impact of frontline staff working with the exceptionally high volume of critically ill patients had been recognised, and HEE (2020b) published *Healthcare Learners Coronavirus Advice Guide* and provided information about recognising burnout and stress factors in the 'Wellbeing and Self Care' section.

Achieving Annexe B proficiencies

Despite the academic challenges of online learning and student experience, a growing concern in this maelstrom of clinical practice was the students' ability to achieve some of the Annexe B proficiencies. Even before lockdown it was apparent there were going to be challenges, not least because of the hesitancy from some clinical placement areas to revise their policies to permit students to engage in the more advanced clinical skills. As an example, there was delay in students achieving proficiency 5.6: *Insert, manage and remove oral/nasal and gastric tubes.* BAPEN (British Association for Parenteral and Enteral Nutrition) had published a position paper prepared by the Nasogastric Tube Specialist Group (BAPEN, 2020) where it was stated they strongly supported restriction of nasogastric tube insertion to registered nurses. Therefore, amendment of a policy which permitted student nurses to insert nasogastric tubes could be regarded as flying the face of a professional recommendation.

Equally concerning was the absence of appropriate clinical opportunity in some instances. In another example, nursing students in the fields of mental health and learning disability were unlikely to have the experience of cannulating patients in clinical practice and not all registered nurses were themselves skilled in some of the required proficiencies. The immediacy of the problem was such that third year students nearing the end of their course could potentially experience a delay in completing and registering with the NMC. The concern was that any delay would negatively impact on workforce recruitment at a time when NHS staff shortages were at a critical point. A possible solution was found through simulated and virtual learning (SIM) within the university settings.

The NMC in their Current Emergency and Recovery Programme Standards (NMC, 2021) permitted a maximum of 300 hours of SIM to be used as part of the legislated standard of a minimum of 2300 practice hours, although there was also the stipulation that the final placement for third year students should take place *'in an audited practice placement setting'.* As with digital technologies, SIM had been evolving over a similar time frame and for the first time, not only could it be counted toward practice hours, but students could also be assessed in this virtual environment. Historically SIM had been the approach used to teach clinical skills and for students to practise them, but now the Student Supervision and Assessment framework (NMC, 2018a) allowed for proficiencies to be assessed and signed off as 'achieved' in the virtual environment. By summer 2020, this timely intervention coincided with university simulation facilities beginning to re-open, albeit with reduced student numbers, in line with the mandated Covid-19 requirement for social distancing and use of personal protective equipment.

However, as progress was being made in assessing proficiencies, there was a more mundane but nevertheless crucial issue emerging for those universities who had not yet transferred over to electronic practice assessment documentation (e-PAD). As students completed a 'stage', their hard copy PAD had to be submitted for marking and confirmation of progression. Logistically, this now was extremely challenging. There was no university facility for students to hand in their PADs, so instead they relied on scanning each page onto a digital platform, which was typically via the cameras on their phones. Lecturers often found marking in this format difficult when pages were presented at a variety of angles. Furthermore, arranging for new PADs to be printed and distributed to students was a logistical nightmare, not least because it all had to be managed by staff working from home who were tasked to ensure the right PAD was sent to the right student at the right address in time for the start of their placement.

The advantages of e-PADs were already understood and the lockdown scenario provided an immediate solution to the problems of communication between academic assessors and practice assessors and supervisors. The emergency standards (NMC, 2020b) had amalgamated the roles of the practice assessor and practice supervisor in order to streamline the assessment process, but despite these measures, the unprecedented clinical pressures were not always conducive to easy communication between the two assessor roles, a situation compounded further by the inability of academic assessors to visit clinical areas during lockdown; they were therefore wholly reliant on telephone or digital communication channels with practice staff and their students.

As digital communication extends across nurse education and mainstream clinical care, consideration needs to be given to how it interplays with student placements. This is in particular reference to the expectation that nurses must be able to care for people in their own homes and in the community (NMC, 2018a) and therefore need the experience of community-based placements to achieve these skills. Prior to the pandemic there was a shortage of appropriate audited placements but the impact of Covid-19 has further significantly reduced placement capacity, especially in the community setting. Pre-existing low staff ratios, current staff sickness and concerns for staff, student and patient safety have contributed to the decline in capacity but so too has the policy adopted by some primary care providers that does not permit students to car share with their community nurses during lockdown. As only very few students own cars, their only opportunity for a community placement was via a digital platform to facilitate their engagement with patients or service users and practice assessors. While the availability of a virtual, digitally enhanced placement was helpful for a limited number of students, it also had obvious disadvantages when it came to achieving some clinically specific Annexe B proficiencies. However, throughout the Covid-19 pandemic, the use of digital and simulation technologies undoubtedly kept the practice education wheels moving. The question is how nurse education will take forward what in the first instance was a pragmatic short-term solution in the long term.

Next steps

Pre-registration nursing education was intentionally going to be transformed by the NMC (2018a) *Future Nurse* standards, but no one could have envisaged the subsequent influence of the pandemic. The accelerated move to online learning was essential but as pandemic restrictions slowly subside and students are gradually returning to face-to-face teaching, there still needs to be recognition of the 'digital divide' between the poorest and most affluent students, and its subsequent impact on their learning (Haslam, 2020). The investment in digital platforms and overall benefits to student learning means that it is likely that online learning will continue to have an integral position in nurse education, so perhaps this is the time universities need to consider students' home-based accessibility to digital technology including internet connectivity.

It is possible that, as well as being disruptive, Covid-19 could be viewed as a positive agent of change, or at least this may be the case when considering the conundrum of clinical placement capacity. Aside from utilising SIM as a placement equivalent, Carolan et al (2020) suggest that online learning offers an opportunity to shift away from the traditional separation of theory and practice 'blocks' to running them in parallel instead, as happens in Australia. Students would be accessing online learning materials when concurrently they would also be in clinical practice. This is not dissimilar to how many post-registration courses are facilitated and the advantages are that students would not have to endure long periods of social isolation in a theory block; they would be able to practise their clinical skills learnt in SIM and this could also overcome many of the timetabling challenges of finding placements for students who have had to temporarily defer the course (an issue that Covid-19 has magnified exponentially), because appropriate placements will be allocated as they become available rather than working to an exact practice placement timetable.

Lastly, Covid-19 has impacted upon the practice learning experience of pre-registration nursing students, but this can be viewed just as easily as an unprecedented opportunity to be grasped by nurse educators and practice partners alike to embrace change for the benefit of the future workforce.

Reflective questions

» Is it possible for all four fields of pre-registration nursing students to successfully achieve Annexe B proficiencies in a clinical practice environment without reliance on SIM?

» How may parity be achieved for all students to access the digital technology necessary for online learning?

» How may the challenges of placement capacity be overcome? To what extent can this be influenced by NMC directives on placement hours and by rethinking theory and practice timetables?

References

BAPEN (2020) *A Position Paper on Nasogastric Tube Safety: 'Time to put patient safety first'*. Prepared by the NGSIG (Nasogastric Tube Special Interest Group of BAPEN). [online] Available at: www.bapen.org.uk/pdfs/ngsig/a-position-paper-on-nasogastric-tube-safety.pdf (accessed 3 January 2022).

Barker, K, Omoni, G, Wakasiaka, S, Watiti, J, Mathai, M and Lavender, T (2013) 'Moving with the Times' – Taking a Global Approach: A Qualitative Study of African Student Nurse Views of e-Learning. *Nurse Education Today*, 33(4): 407–12. https://doi.org/10.1016/j.nedt.2013.001.

Bramer, C (2020) Preregistration Adult Nursing Students' Experience of Online Learning: A Qualitative Study. *British Journal of Nursing*, 29(12): 677–83. https://doi.org/10.12968/bjon.2020.29.12.677.

Carolan C, Davies C, Crookes P and McGhee, S (2020) COVID-19: Disruptive Impacts and Transformative Opportunities in Undergraduate Nurse Education. *Nurse Education in Practice*, 46: 1102807. https://doi.org/j.nepr.2020.102807.

Haslam, C (2020) Aging, Connectedness and COVID: An Excerpt from 'Together Apart'. [online] Available at: www.socialsciencespace.com/2020/07/aging-connectedness-and-covid-an-excerpt-from-together-apart/ (accessed 1 August 2021).

Health Education England (2020a) Student Support Guidance During COVID-19 Outbreak. [online] Available at: www.hee.nhs.uk/sites/default/files/documents/Student%20support%20guide%20master%20.pdf (accessed 5 August 2021).

Health Education England (2020b) Healthcare Learners Coronavirus Advice Guide. [online] Available at: https://skillsforhealth.org.uk/wp-content/uploads/2021/01/HealthcareLearnersCovid-19AdviceGuide_Final2.pdf (accessed 5 August 2021).

Nursing and Midwifery Council (2008) *Standards to Support Learning and Assessment in Practice.* NMC standards for mentors, practice teachers and teachers. London: Nursing and Midwifery Council.

Nursing and Midwifery Council (2018a) *Future Nurse: Standards of Proficiency for Registered Nurses.* London: Nursing and Midwifery Council.

Nursing and Midwifery Council (2018b) *Realising Professionalism. Standards for Education and Training. Part 2: Standards for Student Supervision and Assessment.* London: Nursing and Midwifery Council.

Nursing and Midwifery Council (2018c) *The Code. Professional Standards of Practice and Behaviour for Nurses, Midwives and Nursing Associates.* London: Nursing and Midwifery Council.

Nursing and Midwifery Council (2020a) *NMC Response to the Covid-19 Emergency.* London: Nursing and Midwifery Council.

Nursing and Midwifery Council (2020b) *Emergency Standards for Nursing and Midwifery Education.* London: Nursing and Midwifery Council.

Nursing and Midwifery Council (2021) Current Emergency and Recovery Programme Standards. [online] Available at: www.nmc.org.uk/globalassets/sitedocuments/education-standards/current-recovery-programme-standards.pdf (accessed 6 August 2021).

NHS (2019) The NHS Long Term Plan. [online] Available at: www.longtermplan.nhs.uk (accessed 3 January 2022).

O'Gorman, J, Ion, R and Burnett, A (2020) Is this a First Step Towards Treating Students as Equals? *Nursing Standard*, 35(9): 31–2. doi:10.7748/ns.35.9.31.s14.

Smith, G, Passmore, D and Faught, T (2009) The Challenges of Online Nursing Education. *Nurse Education Today*, 12(2): 98–103.

Taft, S H, Perkowski, T and Martin, L S (2011) A Framework for Evaluating Class Size in Online Education. *Quarterly Review of Distance Education*, 12(3): 181–97. https://oaks.kent.edu/node/3614.

Webb, L, Clough, J, O'Reilly, D, Wilmott, D and Witham, G (2017) The Utility and Impact of Information Communication Technology (ICT) for Pre-Registration Nurse Education: A Narrative Synthesis Systematic Review. *Nurse Education Today*, 48: 160–71. https://doi.org/10.1016/j.nedt.2016.10.007.

Chapter 4 | Covid-19 and the virtual generation

Sarah Anderson, Cheryl Bardell, Abigail Doe, Emma Grady, Chloe Harrison, David Healey, Toritseju K Imewe, Peter McNally, Lydia Nambe and Karen Skinner (BASW students)

Who we are: as a group, we are the team behind the British Association of Social Workers (BASW) students' Twitter account. We manage and maintain the Twitter account voluntarily and we are all student members of BASW. Our team consists of social work students from across the UK. We came together virtually through the social media platform Twitter. We all shared a newfound interest in using social media, primarily through the Covid-19 pandemic, and had a collective desire to meet students from different parts of the UK. The BASW students' Twitter account provides a central point for student BASW members from across the UK to discover everything that BASW has to offer, such as continuing professional development (CPD), training, events and networking opportunities. It was from this initiative that we found friendships which would never have evolved if it had not been for social media during Covid-19. We have supported each other during our transition as part of the 'virtual generation' of student social workers.

Introduction

Globally, the Covid-19 pandemic has impacted immensely on how people live their day-to-day lives. As members of a people profession, social work students must learn to work alongside individuals and families, empowering and supporting them to overcome any challenges they may face. But how does a student learn the skills and knowledge required to be a social worker when the most fundamental aspects of social work, people and relationships, are all changed almost overnight?

In this chapter we discuss what have been our most prominent learning curves, challenges and positive outcomes from the past 18 months, since the first UK lockdown in March 2020. We have chosen to explore and reflect on our own experiences of learning, access, well-being and placements during this time.

What is apparent through our reflections is that Covid-19 has changed the course of our social work journeys. What we may have originally envisaged as our social work education could not be further from the reality in the year 2021. It is our hope that this chapter reflects how we have overcome some of these challenges and embraced new ways of learning and practice.

For us as authors, what has been most interesting about writing this chapter is discovering our great diversity as individuals and how unique our journeys into social work are. Although we are from different parts of the UK, we all have similarities and common experiences that describe our student social work journey so far through the Covid-19 pandemic. This sharing is reflected in the way we have structured this chapter. With ten of us involved as authors, we have divided up the work so that everyone's voice is reflected within the chapter.

Learning

This past academic year has been full of twists and turns which have caused many issues for social work students. As TJ, Chloe, Emma and David reflect here, adapting to virtual learning has been constantly challenging.

Some students were lucky enough to experience face-to-face learning at the start of the pandemic, but only for a short while. This taster of face-to-face learning was encouraging although short lived. Unfortunately for most students, face-to-face learning would very quickly be a thing of the past.

Virtual learning is not suitable for everyone, although it can also be advantageous for many. As student author Emma describes, she has found her grades have improved and her ability to concentrate has greatly increased by working in her home environment, but this has not come without its challenges. We soon discovered there were concerns around the cost of virtual learning – for example, the compatibility of a laptop or computer with now required applications such as video calls. Chloe questions whether students could afford adequate broadband packages with speeds that support virtual learning or if it is possible to be in a suitable environment to engage fully with lecturers. Perhaps there are children at home or other distractions that may impact on the ability of students to absorb information and actively engage in lessons.

This also raised the question around the suitability of online learning for students living with attention deficit hyperactivity disorder (ADHD), attention deficit disorder (ADD) or dyslexia. As students, we recognise most lessons are in a standard format and may not consider individual learning needs. We also discovered that many universities are using different approaches to manage the impact of Covid-19 and virtual learning, which may lead to inconsistencies in the delivery of social work education.

Some universities appear to be more adaptive and forward thinking than others, possibly resulting in disparities in social work education (Mitchell and Mawn, 2021).

However, we discussed the advantages of virtual learning and the benefits of spending more time in our home environments – for example, the potential savings on childcare costs and the positive aspect of spending more time with our children and families. For some it could be argued that the work–life balance has been restored. Similarly, reduced travel costs are also an important factor for some students who previously had significant journeys to get to university, plus the positive aspect of not having long journeys can improve mood and well-being.

Technological advances have also made it easier to keep in touch with others (Renu, 2021). Smartphone applications such as WhatsApp, Facebook Messenger and Google Meet or Microsoft Teams allow students to come together at convenient times to chat or discuss lessons and assignment briefs, although we are also aware of some of the privacy arguments around these activities. Online learning may also offer a safe learning space in an environment which can reduce anxieties and stress for those who lack confidence in the classroom.

From our discussions as a group, it became clear that we all have different views on the positive and negative aspects of this past 18 months, but we do agree that it has given us new skills and ways of accomplishing our goals which we would never have previously expected.

Access to learning

Access to learning during Covid-19 is a contested topic which goes much further than home versus campus learning, as Sarah, David and Abigail reflect.

Sarah is a student who worries about returning to 'normal' and on campus learning. As a student with several disabilities, Sarah worries about being among other classmates and colleagues during the Covid-19 pandemic, which could potentially compromise her health (Maben and Bridges, 2020). Sarah is also anxious about the availability of suitable furniture, the suitability of campus bathrooms and the exhaustion of commuting to and from university. Consequently, students like Sarah have greatly benefited from home learning, taking part in extracurricular activities to bridge knowledge gaps and make friends, as well as the flexibility of studying when health allowed, meaning that she and other students can take greater ownership of how and when they learn. This would not have been a possibility before the Covid-19 lockdowns. Sarah is also greatly impacted by low energy levels and individual care needs when out and about on campus, therefore she worries about being marked absent or struggling to get to class on time when she feels ill.

Sarah recognises the possible disadvantages of home learning, including the appropriateness of discussing sensitive topics in a shared environment. As a student representative Sarah also recognises the importance of choice for students in determining their preferred individual learning style (Whalley et al, 2021).

Abigail is also a student representative for the master's group and is aware of student concerns regarding access to library resources, whether in person or virtually. This includes worries about shouldering the financial burdens of buying expensive books, as well as the availability of books in the library. Abigail has found lecturers to be responsive to emails; some students, however, occasionally perceive their responses as vague. Abigail recognises the ease of face-to-face conversation, where questions that may take a day or two to get a response by email could have been answered or followed up more effectively in person (Intening, 2021).

Technology remains a constant worry, as some students do not have access to a laptop at home and if the campus library is closed, how then can a student manage? Abigail found access to lecture transcripts beneficial, but these could be less useful where subtitles are incorrect. Abigail acknowledges that the positions and current circumstances of students are all unique and individual, and at times individual financial situations can play a huge part in students' ability to access quality learning (Chatterjee and Chakraborty, 2020).

David, another social work student author, also recognises the importance of adaptability and believes we need to try to both manage and where possible overcome any difficult situations that cross our paths, including the Covid-19 pandemic. David emphasises his own response to the challenges of the last academic year, where he has been forced to switch to virtual learning and seek out his own ways to replace face-to-face conversations. David recognises the importance of social connections when in the university environment and recalls the benefits of face-to-face support and guidance. There is something special about interacting with your peers and classmates, sharing highs and lows face-to-face. Perhaps now David sees this as special, when once we would have classed it as 'normal' (Son et al, 2020). Something which David has reflected on is access to lecturers and staff members. Being physically present helps with active engagement, where, for example, knowledge can be embedded through the spontaneous asking of questions and receiving of feedback. David feels this is much more difficult online due to distance and the impersonal nature of virtual learning, where there is the capacity to switch off cameras and microphones (Intening, 2021).

Confidence is sometimes an area where students struggle within groups and virtual learning can also remove the anxieties or stress of being present with others. Students can feel invisible in large groups and can often feel as if they don't have a voice. However, through virtual learning some students can build their confidence in their own environment, taking forward these skills into their education.

Campus versus virtual learning is complex, hence we agreed that personal choice is paramount during Covid-19 and hopefully thereafter. Students have genuine reasons to prefer one style over another, or a mixture of both. To ensure future social workers are diverse and dynamic we suggest enabling choice is positive and may perhaps encourage greater participation from people from marginalised backgrounds, where traditional learning may not be a possibility.

Well-being

Sarah has post-traumatic stress disorder (PTSD) caused by sepsis and has chosen to study social work due to lived experience. Sarah isolated before the first national lockdown, as she is immunocompromised. This caused rapid mental health decline and evoked feelings of worry about access to prescriptions and groceries, no outside space and aggravated flashbacks due to being vulnerable (Son et al, 2020). These anxieties reached a point where her mental health became so precarious that her parents asked that she return home. This allowed her garden access, although there were stressors with shared living space. Sarah reflects and acknowledges the well-being inequalities, when access to facilities such as green spaces is limited, a situation also shared by classmates who were isolating in halls. Sarah urges that self-care is written into social work teaching with practical suggestions which could be used during employment to enhance resilience and prevent burnout (Ku and Brantley, 2020).

Concerns surrounding self-care are also shared by Karen. Karen reflects on her own experiences of mental ill health and she believes Covid-19 has highlighted the importance of resilience as we try to balance the arduous tasks of managing the impact of the pandemic, looking after our mental health, studying, working and being part of a family. Karen recognises the negative impact of not travelling to and from places of work and education, as for many this can be a time to reflect and de-stress.

Karen believes practical methods should be encouraged in social work including meditation and mindfulness within the classroom which may have a positive impact on student and newly qualified social worker (NQSW) well-being. She believes universities should be proactive in team building, as students may find it challenging and emotionally draining discussing highly emotive subjects with individuals they have never met before. Karen recognises the challenges of building relationships with her cohort where in many cases, virtual learning has prevented any actual face-to-face meetings (Browning et al, 2021).

Social work students are given opportunities to discuss and reflect on the intersection between personal and social issues (QAA, 2019, p 10). The topics tend to be serious and emotive. For example, Abigail completed an assignment on individual issues with links to social problems. The work was reflexive and affected her mental health, as she reflected on a hurtful memory. Abigail tried various techniques to help with her mental well-being, such as self-help audiobooks, breathing exercises and a meditation app recommended by her university's mental health support service. She overcame this turbulent time by reframing her thinking and beliefs to positive goal-oriented action based on her values using Adlerian psychotherapy (Kishimi and Koga, 2018). Adlerian psychotherapy provides a remedy for an individual's self-perceived inferiority based on the strengths of individuals and the interpersonal relationship with others (Belangee, 2019).

Abigail believes that universities should reassure students that good well-being enhances learning while completing their education (Social Work England, 2021). Students should be encouraged by their universities to take adequate time off, if required, without them feeling the urge to bounce back quickly from a mentally challenging life episode.

Placements

Placements are a crucial part of any social work programme. While some students experienced face-to-face placements, for many they were cancelled, postponed or switched to virtual placements. In this section Lydia and Cheryl reflect on their experiences of placements during the Covid-19 pandemic.

For Cheryl, the thought of having a virtual placement initially caused some anxieties. However, recently reflecting on the experience, it is apparent that it has provided learning opportunities that may not have been so readily available in a face-to-face placement. Having a virtual placement allows the student to begin to become a 'digital resident' (White and Le Cornu, 2011). The use of applications such as Zoom and Microsoft Teams provides the platform from which to acquire skills and develop digital capabilities in providing support and delivering interventions to service users online. It is important to remain mindful that not all service users will have easy access to technology, for example, due to disability or not being able to afford devices and internet connection. A strength of having a virtual placement is that it encourages the use of new and creative ways to engage with service users.

While a common concern about having a virtual placement is that it might limit the opportunities to shadow experienced practitioners, in some settings the opposite is true. With practitioners working from home, arranging to 'listen in' on calls to service users and professionals from different agencies, with consent, may be easier. Also, while experienced practitioners adjust to these newer ways of working there may be opportunities for them to learn from students about the resources, ways of delivering interventions and skills that they have developed during placement.

Lydia recalls the words of her first lecturer: *'relationships are the cornerstone of social work',* and Lydia reflects upon these words as she discusses her previous placement. For effective social work practice, the quality of the relationship between the practitioner and service user is central (Department of Health, 2017). During Lydia's placement in a child and family team, she observed interactions, which led to a deep understanding of the complex dynamics in relationships. Lydia noticed the relationships between parents and children during family time or in their home, the relationships professionals have with parents and carers, even the relationships parents have with each other, observing high levels of trauma in these relationships, amplified by the pandemic.

While on placement Lydia also examined the relationships with the children, parents and carers with whom she worked, her team, other professionals, her supervisor, and practice educator. She concluded that the most important relationship is the one she has with herself, highlighting the need to continuously reflect on her actions and interactions to know her limitations, strengths and biases. She realised from her placement experiences that even as a student, her actions and words impact on other lives, hence the necessity to be trauma-aware, ensuring she is acting compassionately and using her role on placement in the most effective way. Lydia believes she must treat the people who encounter her with compassion, but most importantly treat herself with compassion to ensure she can become the best social worker she can be.

Conclusion

It could be argued that social work education will never go back to how it was before March 2020. The Covid-19 pandemic has impacted every human being in ways that we could never have imagined. If anything, the past 18 months have shown the commitment, resilience, diligence and willpower of all students involved to succeed. The social work education journey has been difficult, and every student has experienced the lockdown in different ways. Yet all students have shown that the human spirit will always adapt to challenges set out for them.

Social work is about people and being 'social', yet we have been more confined to computers than ever before. We have been further 'away' from people than ever before, yet we have been brought closer to people we never thought we would reach. Mental health, well-being and personal reflection have perhaps never been as important as they are now, and perhaps as we adapt to the 'new-normal' we will also adapt to working more on ourselves, our priorities, our happiness, well-being and mental health – after all, if we don't invest in ourselves, how can we invest in those who need us most?

Reflective questions

» As students do we really want to return to 'normal'?

» Is the new virtual generation the 'new normal'?

» Should we be seeking more ways to offer choice in learning styles for all students to make education more accessible?

References

Belangee, S (2019) Adlerian Psychology in the Era of Evidence-Based Practice: A Reflection from a Clinician in Private Practice. *The Journal of Individual Psychology* (1998), 75(3): 205–9. doi:10.1353/jip.2019.0026.

Browning, M, Larson, L, Sharaievska, I, Rigolon, A, McAnirlin, O, Mullenbach, L, Cloutier, S, Vu, T, Thomsen, J, Reigner, N, Metcalf, E, D'Antonio, A, Helbich, M, Bratman, G and Alvarez, H (2021) Psychological Impacts from COVID-19 Among University Students: Risk Factors Across Seven States in the United States. *PLOS ONE*, 16(1): e0245327.

Chatterjee, I and Chakraborty, P (2020) Use of Information Communication Technology by Medical Educators Amid COVID-19 Pandemic and Beyond. *Journal of Educational Technology Systems*, 49(3): 310–24.

Department of Health (2017) *The Purpose of Social Work Improvement and Safeguarding Social Wellbeing.* Belfast: Department of Health.

Intening, V (2021) The Lecturers and Students Satisfaction in Conducting Online Learning During Covid-19 Pandemic. *Journal Kesehatan*, 8(2): 131–7.

Kishimi, I and Koga, F (2018) *The Courage to Be Disliked: How to Free Yourself, Change Your Life and Achieve Real Happiness.* Worldwide: Allen and Unwin.

Ku, L and Brantley, E (2020) Widening Social and Health Inequalities During the COVID-19 Pandemic. *JAMA Health Forum*, 1(6): e200721.

Maben, J and Bridges, J (2020) Covid-19: Supporting Nurses' Psychological and Mental Health. *Journal of Clinical Nursing*, 29(15–16): 2742–50.

Mitchell, R and Mawn, C (2021) Thinking the Unthinkable to Support Students in this Third Lockdown. *Community Care*, 6 January. [online] Available at: www.communitycare.co.uk/2021/01/06/future-social-work-impact-pandemic-students/ (accessed 3 January 2022).

Quality Assurance Agency for UK Higher Education (QAA) (2019) *Subject Benchmark Statement.* [online] Available at: www.qaa.ac.uk/docs/qaa/subject-benchmark-statements/subject-benchmark-statement-social-work.pdf?sfvrsn=5c35c881/ (accessed 13 January 2022).

Renu, N (2021) Technological Advancement in the Era of COVID-19. *SAGE Open Medicine*, 9: 205031212110009.

Social Work England (2021) *Qualifying Education and Training Standards Guidance 2021.* [online] Available at: www.socialworkengland.org.uk/standards/qualifying-education-and-training-standards-guidance-2021/ (accessed 3 January 2022).

Son, C, Hegde, S, Smith, A, Wang, X and Sasangohar, F (2020) Effects of COVID-19 on College Students' Mental Health in the United States: Interview Survey Study. *Journal of Medical Internet Research*, 22(9): e21279.

Whalley, B, France, D, Park, J, Mauchline, A and Welsh, K (2021) Towards Flexible Personalized Learning and the Future Educational System in the Fourth Industrial Revolution in the Wake of Covid-19. *Higher Education Pedagogies*, 6(1): 79–99.

White, D S and Le Cornu, A (2011) Visitors and Residents: A New Typology for Engagement. *First Monday*, 16(9). [online] Available at: http://firstmonday.org/ojs/index.php/fm/article/view/3171/3049 (accessed 3 January 2022).

Chapter 5 | 'I am not a cat': Digital capabilities and Covid-19

Dr Denise Turner

Introduction

With the growth of the Web 2.0 generation (Kaplan and Haenlein, 2010, p 61) the role of digital technology in our public and personal lives has been more hotly debated than ever before. Much of the debate centres around the threats posed by online technologies through data collection and cyber-crime (Goldkind et al, 2020; Bossler and Berenblum, 2019), while potential relational damage has also been the subject of scrutiny. For example, in her influential book *Alone Together*, Turkle (2011, p 1) argues that *'the connected life encourages us to treat those we meet online in something of the same way we treat objects – with dispatch'*. However, since the imposition of the global Covid-19 pandemic, 'the connected life' has been the only way that much of the global population has maintained any form of work or personal relationships. While this has raised many challenges, not least for those without technological resources, there have also been multiple opportunities to run campaigns and develop virtual communities which have helped disparate groups to connect and find support during the crisis.

This chapter explores some of the significant digital opportunities, as well as the challenges, resulting from the Covid-19 pandemic, via the three main domains of the Digital Capabilities for Social Workers statement (SCIE, 2020; BASW, 2020a). Fatefully, this statement was published in March 2020, at the same time as the first UK lockdown, thereby providing an unexpected opportunity for live trialling, as social work education and practice moved rapidly online.

Digital capabilities for social work

The Digital Capabilities project was commissioned by Health Education England in 2019 as part of the Building a Digitally Ready Workforce programme. The project was supported by NHS Digital and delivered by both the British Association of Social Workers (BASW) and the Social Care Institute for Excellence (SCIE), with the aim of helping social workers and stakeholders to develop and enhance their online skills.

Preliminary research for the project (Turner, 2019) found that only a small minority of social workers felt that they were 'digitally ready' for undertaking their work. Continuing professional development (CPD) in the form of in-work training and development opportunities were also very rare, with only 27 per cent of respondents in the research receiving any training in the previous two years. Significantly for social work education, only a very small sample of participants in the research believed that their initial social work training had prepared them for being digitally competent or capable in practice, while over half had found their training actively unhelpful (Turner, 2019).

The Digital Capabilities project reported in March 2020, at the same time as the UK was pitched into the first national lockdown. Included among the project's key outputs were a set of resources, including the Digital Capabilities statement, which provides a framework for the skills and values that social workers require in order to practise digitally with children and adults, as well as adhering to both professional and regulatory standards. The statement is divided into three key domains – purpose, practice and impact – which this chapter seeks to explore through practice examples drawn from the pandemic.

Purpose

Alongside early critics of digital connectivity (Turkle, 2011), social work as a profession has also occupied an ambivalent position in relation to increasing digitisation (Taylor-Beswick, 2019). Despite this, there have been many digital pioneers within social work (LaMendola, 1985; Rafferty, 1996; Sapey, 1997) and issues of technology were being debated as long ago as the 1970s (Taylor-Beswick, 2021). Nevertheless, digital adoption within the profession has been slow and often treated with suspicion and reluctance (Turner, 2016), an attitude which accounts for the preliminary findings of the Digital Capabilities project (SCIE, 2020; BASW, 2020a). As a result of this, and long before Covid-19, Baker et al (2014, p 468) gave a prescient rallying call for social work to 'overcome its historical reluctance to embrace ICT if it is to remain relevant in the era of the networked society'.

This ambivalent and sometimes even resistant relationship with technology is reflected in the initial question posed within the purpose section of the digital capabilities statement: 'Why should social workers develop their digital capabilities?' (SCIE, 2020; BASW, 2020a). The Covid-19 pandemic and accompanying uptake of digital resources across personal and public life have provided a resounding answer to this question. In practice, social workers suddenly found themselves contacting parents through WhatsApp, Zoom and other video enabled platforms, with accompanying feelings of 'anxiety and helplessness' (Labuschagne et al, 2021, p 15). Correspondingly, in social work education, students and academics were catapulted onto previously unexplored platforms, proving irrefutably the need for digital capability. In this sudden and unexpected online environment, new opportunities for cyber-crime and data extraction were also generated, rendering knowledge and understanding of the risks associated with big data a vital skill for social work educators and practitioners alike (Goldkind et al, 2020; Zetino and Mendoza, 2019).

Alongside knowledge of digital platforms and the potential risks associated with these, two other crucial points within the purpose domain of the digital capabilities statement were highlighted by the lockdowns. The framework recommends that social workers learn 'how to use digital technologies to enhance face-to-face contact', as well as directing people to online services and networks which can 'reduce loneliness, provide therapeutic interventions and enhance peoples' community networks' (SCIE, 2020; BASW, 2020a).

Considering that these findings pre-date the pandemic, they are particularly prescient, since the repeated series of lockdowns since March 2020 are known to have increased loneliness and amplified mental health issues within the UK population. Evidence from Public Health England (2021) suggests that mental health and wellbeing deteriorated rapidly during the first national lockdown in March 2020, with signs of an improvement once the lockdown was lifted in July that year. Mental health issues then deteriorated again in the winter of 2020 as new variants of the virus were discovered and restrictions re-imposed. Significantly for social work, some of the most recent findings from Public Health England (2021) show that particular attention needs to be paid to vulnerable groups, making the recommendations of the digital capabilities statement – that social workers harness digital technologies to reduce loneliness – particularly pressing.

Practice

The practice domain of the digital capabilities statement presciently states that social workers should 'understand the online uses and technology needs of people who use services', with particular reference to use of technology 'to support their wellbeing' (SCIE, 2020; BASW, 2020a), a concern that has increased during Covid-19 due to repeated lockdowns, multiple losses and social isolation.

Writing over a decade before the Covid-19 pandemic, boyd (2013) coined the term 'collapsed contexts' which later evolved into the popular term, 'context collapse' (Marwick and boyd, 2010) to describe ways in which boundaries have been disrupted by the digital world. The Covid-19 pandemic has suddenly animated this 'context collapse' in previously unimaginable ways, as office, home, school and university all became folded into one. Domestic violence has soared, as people have been forced together in often cramped or unsuitable living spaces, with concomitant effects on children and warnings of a *second pandemic* in the form of increased child abuse and neglect (Øverlien, 2020, p 1). Home schooling has been shown to have potentially detrimental impacts, particularly on mothers (Petts et al, 2021), while 'digital exclusion' has also precluded whole sections of the population from connecting with their personal and professional networks (Watling, 2011).

For a fortunate few, total 'context collapse' could be avoided through use of a study or dedicated work area, but for many there was only the kitchen table, or tiny areas of already cramped accommodation. Sentamu, a Ugandan social work student, describes this vividly in his account of experiencing 'severe symptoms of Covid-19' while living with three children and his partner in a two-bedroom flat: *'The available bedroom for self-isolation had very poor internet access which greatly hindered [my] ability to access online materials for studying'* (Sentamu, p 55, cited in Lorimer et al, 2021).

The 'context collapse' created by Covid-19, while presenting significant challenges to well-being, as documented by Sentamu (Lorimer et al, 2021) also arguably introduced an accompanying venue versatility, with the flourishing of multiple online initiatives which testify to this (Health in Mind, nd; Healthline, 2021). #Starsinmemory, a campaign run by the National Care Forum (NCF) and National Activity Providers Association (NAPA) in June 2020, provided a national opportunity for people across the UK to remember those that had died as a result of the pandemic by creating a star and placing it in their window, or by using the hashtag on social media (National Care Forum, 2020). The project, which united over 30 care organisations, was devised, developed and delivered entirely online, with hundreds of organisations posting to social media, thereby testifying to the power of technology in unifying people (*Huffington Post*, 2020). A similar project, #Momentintime21, held in July 2021, invited people to create a time capsule to share memories of the pandemic, with all the development and resources similarly delivered entirely through online community interaction (National Care Forum, 2021; *The Carer*, 2021).

On a more personal level, the simultaneous, enforced move online for such a large proportion of the population has also generated creativity and community in the use of online platforms. Taylor (2021, p 69) describes powerfully being a *'disabled person'* within the pandemic, with much of her well-being dependent on connecting with and supporting others through a *'community social app'*. For Taylor, these online connections provided some of the most meaningful moments of her pandemic experiences (Turner, 2016).

During the early part of the Covid-19 pandemic, the venue versatility offered by digital platforms was also demonstrated through the creation of a digital social work community, 'Connecting Social Work During Social Isolation' (BASW, 2020b) using the online facility Padlet. Simple and accessible in design, Padlet offers an online bulletin board into which audio, video, images and text can be embedded, thereby allowing for easy online connection. The wall established during the first lockdown aimed specifically at reducing isolation and rapidly became an abundant source of sharing, as well as 'escapism' from the rigours of social distancing and estrangement from pre-pandemic life (Lorimer et al, 2021). As the weeks passed, multiple contributors to this Padlet community began to post regular photographs of wildlife encountered on their one permitted walk a day, while a community of poetry lovers also began to evolve. Starting with a few postings about poetry and some selected verse, this emerging community has gone on to build nationwide networks through poetry workshops from London to Scotland, once again demonstrating the potential power of online connection for enhancing well-being.

The Padlet community, formed through the first lockdown, became a vivid testimony to the practice domain in the digital capabilities project which calls for social workers to use technology to *'support ... wellbeing'* (SCIE, 2020), with one student contributor summarising this powerfully: *'Padlet helped [me] to find humanity again'* (Sharples, p 57, cited in Lorimer et al, 2021).

However, regardless of the many positive opportunities afforded by technology during the pandemic, another key point highlighted by the practice domain of the digital capabilities statement is the necessity for social workers to embrace ethical decision making and maintain data security. This is particularly significant given the large amount of personal information which social workers can access, as well as the risk of 'boundary issues' (SCIE, 2020; BASW, 2020a). The pandemic has exacerbated these issues and, as Goldkind et al (2020, p 89) suggest, tackling these consequently requires some urgency since *'a significant portion of the general public is now reliant on digital tools that have not fully considered user privacy'*. Using Zoom as an example, the authors argue that *'this is a major corporate body with little or no oversight'* which fails to offer significant protection for vulnerable service users. Secara (2020, p 1) also writes of the phenomenon of *'Zoom bombing a practice of gate-crashing online conferences and other groups, which began as a prank, but rapidly migrated to organised targeting with pornographic and/or hate images and threatening language'*.

Aside from such organised activity, professionalism can be impacted in other ways through the use of online technology in practice. One of the most celebrated examples of this, during the pandemic, occurred during a US court hearing when one of the legal advocates, lawyer Rod Ponton, appeared on screen as a large, fluffy cat. Ponton and his team struggled live to remove the cat filter which had been set by his secretary's daughter but were unable to manage, telling the court: *'I don't know how to remove it. I've got my assistant here, she's trying to, but I'm prepared to go forward with it...I'm here live. I'm not a cat'* (Gabbatt, 2020).

Combined with salient warnings about privacy and big data collection (Goldkind et al, 2020), Ponton's experience serves to highlight one of the key messages in the practice domain of the digital capabilities statement, that *'Social workers need to be able to identify and balance the benefits and the risks of digital technology – and how to miti-gate against those risks'* (SCIE,2020; BASW, 2020a). Additionally, it is vital to consider those who are not able to access the benefits of digital connectivity through digital poverty and other forms of exclusion (Watling, 2011).

Impact

The last key domain of the digital capabilities statement focusses on impact (SCIE, 2020; BASW, 2020a). This includes social work practitioners and educators continu-ally developing and maintaining their digital professionalism, as well as exploring and understanding how online behaviour can affect professional identity – a factor so viv-idly exhibited by Rod Ponton's viral online appearance as a cat (Gabbatt, 2020). As with the previous categories, purpose and practice, impact involves possibilities for positive change, as well as more concerning challenges. Key to both is the necessity for social work educators and practitioners alike to overcome any earlier resistance to technology and to consolidate the skills and competencies acquired through the pan-demic via appropriate CPD activities.

One area for such development which has been powerfully highlighted by Covid-19 is that of *'digital remains'* (Lingel, 2013) arising from the unparalleled death toll since the start of the pandemic. In the UK alone at the time of writing there have been 128,000 deaths from Covid-19, many of which have been sudden and unexpected, with little or no opportunity for advance care planning. Rising smartphone use in the UK, predicted to rise to 93.7 per cent of the population by 2025, means that a large proportion of those who died will have owned a smartphone, or other digital device (Statista, 2020).

This rise in digital ownership is accompanied by complex moral dilemmas for bereaved people and the practitioners who support them. Where once managing someone's estate after death largely involved finances, possibly property and personal effects such as clothes and material goods, the widespread adoption of smartphones and advent of social media platforms such as Facebook and Instagram have created a *'digital graveyard'* (Stokes, 2015) which necessitates convoluted and often highly emotive decision making. For example, should bereaved family and friends have access to someone's digital photos and other online content after death and similarly should they be able to curate social media presence after a person has died? Additionally, the continuing digital presence of someone who has died can complicate grieving for those left behind, leading to prolonged mourning which may require expert professional support (Bell et al, 2015; Kasket, 2012).

Previous research (Turner and Price, 2020) has shown that there is little specific focus on bereavement in social work programmes, nor in CPD.

However, online support sessions carried out with social work practitioners during the pandemic have highlighted a pressing need for greater information and expertise in this area. One group of social work practitioners had experienced the death of several colleagues during the pandemic, when social distancing still precluded the gathering of people for collective mourning. For these practitioners, finding a means of remembering those who had died, despite the restrictions, was a priority for their own well-being. One possible solution, again provided by online technology, was establishing a Padlet memorial wall. Settings for Padlet can be placed on 'private' allowing a measure of confidentiality, while providing an accessible means of collectively remembering those who had died. In this way the simple 'humanity' experienced previously by users of the social work Padlet wall (BASW, 2020b) could be facilitated for this group of bereaved practitioners, despite the ban on collective mourning. Applying such digital solutions creatively to problems created by the pandemic further showcases the possibilities of digital technology for connection and reparation.

The issues raised by *digital remains* (Lingel, 2013) and online mourning have not been widely discussed during the pandemic and remain largely absent from both social work education and CPD. However, these issues powerfully correspond with recommendations within the digital capabilities statement – in particular, the need for social work to keep pace with maintaining digital professionalism over time. With deaths from the pandemic predicted to continue (BBC News, 2021), coping with the ethical and moral implications of 'digital remains' is an important area to consider within the 'impact' of the digital on social work education and practice.

Conclusion

This chapter has explored the three main domains of the digital capabilities statement for social work (SCIE, 2020; BASW, 2020a), connecting these with key issues arising from the Covid-19 pandemic. The purpose domain, which poses the question *'Why should social workers develop their digital capabilities?'*, has been resoundingly answered by a pandemic which has seen millions of people move online for both work and personal connection, often familiarising themselves overnight with previously unfamiliar platforms. The possibilities for connection afforded by digital resources such as Padlet have been discussed, alongside the vital importance of considering ethical issues arising from phenomena such as 'Zoom bombing', data selling, viral work videos and digital exclusion.

Lastly, the phenomenon of 'digital remains' has been discussed with reference to the multiple sudden and unexpected deaths arising from the pandemic. In the UK at the time of writing, there have been over 128,000 deaths and with the lifting of restrictions in July 2019, deaths are predicted to rise to approximately 200 per day (BBC News, 2021). Of these 200 people, most are likely to have a smartphone, some other form of digital device, or social media presence, leaving surviving relatives and friends facing complex moral and ethical choices.

The chapter has aimed to balance these ethical dilemmas as well as the data and privacy concerns with the relational opportunities, which for many have been a lifeline during the Covid-19 pandemic (Turner, 2016). While many of the interventions described within the chapter have been temporary solutions to what appeared in March 2020 to be a similarly transient challenge, as cases continue to multiply in the UK, world leaders are also considering responses to the next pandemic (BBC News, 2021). Against this background, the digital capabilities statement, published concomitantly with the first UK national lockdown, offers an invaluable framework for considering both social work practice and education in an increasingly online world.

Moving forwards into the future, it is vital that learning from the digital capabilities project and from the pandemic itself is consolidated within initial social work education, practice and CPD opportunities.

Reflective questions

» Thinking about the lawyer with the cat filter, what have been your own digital blunders during the pandemic and how have you tried to learn from these?

» What training and other support do you think you need for navigating the complex ethical landscape of online platforms?

» Have you thought about curating your own digital remains?

References

Baker, S, Warburton, J, Hodgkin, S and Pascal, J (2014) Reimagining the Relationship Between Social Work and Information Technology in the Network Society. *Australian Social Work*, 67(4): 467–78.

BASW (2020a) Digital Capabilities Statement for Social Workers. [online] Available at: www.basw.co.uk/digital-capabilities-statement-social-workers (accessed 3 January 2022).

BASW (2020b) Top Tips for Wellbeing: Wellness and Wellbeing Resources for Isolation and Working from Home. [online] Available at: www.basw.co.uk/top-tips-wellbeing (accessed 3 January 2022).

BBC News (2021) Covid-19: World Leaders Call for International Pandemic Treaty. [online] Available at: www.bbc.co.uk/news/uk-56572775 (accessed 10 January 2022).

Bell, J, Bailey, L and Kennedy, D (2015) 'We do it to keep him alive': Bereaved Individuals' Experiences of Online Suicide Memorials and Continuing Bonds. *Mortality*, 20(4): 375–89. doi: 10.1080/13576275.2015.1083693.

Bossler, A and Berenblum, T (2019) Introduction: New Directions in Cybercrime Research. *Journal of Crime and Justice*, 42(5): 495–9. doi: 10.1080/0735648X.2019.1692426,

boyd, d (2013) how 'context collapse' was coined: my recollection. *Apophenia*. [online] Available at: www.zephoria.org/thoughts/archives/2013/12/08/coining-context-collapse.html (accessed 10 January 2022).

Gabbatt, A (2020) Texas Lawyer, Trapped by Cat Filter on Zoom Call, Informs Judge He Is Not a Cat. *The Guardian*. [online] Available at: www.theguardian.com/us-news/2021/feb/09/texas-lawyer-zoom-cat-filter-kitten (accessed 3 January 2022).

Goldkind, L, LaMendola, W and Taylor-Beswick, A (2020) Tackling Covid-19 is a Crucible for Privacy. *Journal of Technology in Human Services*, 38(2): 89–90.

Health in Mind (nd) Moving to Online Support Groups (Covid-19) Blog by Frankie. [online] Available at: www.health-in-mind.org.uk/covid_19_resources/i2278/blog_moving_to_online_support_groups_covid_19.aspx (accessed 10 January 2022).

Healthline (2021) COVID-19 Survivors Share How to Recover During Pandemic. [online] Available at: www.healthline.com/health-news/covid-19-survivors-share-how-to-recover-during-pandemic (accessed 3 January 2022).

Huffington Post (2020) Why People Are Putting Stars In Their Windows As We Come Out Of Lockdown. 30 June. [online] Available at: www.huffingtonpost.co.uk/entry/stars-in-memory-windows-coronavirus_uk_5efb2cb5c5b6acab2846eead (accessed 15 January 2022).

Kaplan, A and Haenlein, M (2010) Users of the World, Unite! The Challenges and Opportunities of Social Media. *Business Horizons*, 53(1): 59–68.

Kasket, E (2012) Being-Towards-Death in the Digital Age. *Existential Analysis: Journal of the Society for Existential Analysis*, 23(2): 249–61.

LaMendola, W (1985) The Future of Human Service Information Technology: An Essay on the Number 42. *Computers in Human Services*, 1(1): 35–49.

Labuschagne, N, Hadridge, G, Vanderbijl, L, Jones, S and Geater, E (2021) Protecting Children during the Pandemic. In Turner, D (ed) *Social Work and Covid-19: Lessons from Education and Practice* (pp 15–22). St Albans: Critical Publishing.

Lingel, J (2013) The Digital Remains: Social Media and Practices of Online Grief. *The Information Society*, 29(3): 190–5.

Lorimer, A Sentamu, F and Sharples, R (2021) From Surviving to Thriving: The Experience of Social Work Students and Their Families in Lockdown. In Turner, D (ed) *Social Work and Covid-19: Lessons from Education and Practice* (pp 53–62). St Albans: Critical Publishing.

Marwick, A and boyd, d (2010) I Tweet Honestly, I Tweet Passionately: Twitter Users, Context Collapse and the Imagined Audience. *New Media and Society*, 13(1): 114–33.

National Care Forum (2020) #StarsInMemory – Connected by Care – United by Loss. [online] Available at: www.nationalcareforum.org.uk/draft/starsinmemory-connected-by-care-united-by-loss/ (accessed 3 January 2022).

National Care Forum (2021) Moment in Time. [online] Available at: www.nationalcareforum.org.uk/moment-in-time/ (accessed 3 January 2022).

Øverlien, C (2020) The COVID-19 Pandemic and Its Impact on Children in Domestic Violence Refuges. *Child Abuse Review*, 29(4): 379–86.

Petts, R J, Carlson, D L and Pepin, J R (2021) A Gendered Pandemic: Childcare, Home Schooling, and Parents' Employment during COVID-19. *Gender Work and Organization*, 28(52): 515–34. doi: 10.1111/gwao.12614.

Public Health England (2021) *Covid-19 Mental Health and Wellbeing Surveillance-Report.* [online] Available at: www.gov.uk/government/publications/covid-19-mental-health-and-wellbeing-surveillance-report/2-important-findings-so-far (accessed 10 January 2022).

Rafferty, J (1996) Learning and Educational Technology in Social Work: Introduction. *Computers in Human Services*, 12(1–2): 69–73.

Sapey, B (1997) Social Work Tomorrow: Towards a Critical Understanding of Technology in Social Work. *The British Journal of Social Work*, 27(6): 802–14.

Secara, I A (2020) Zoom Bombing – The End-to-end Fallacy. *Network Security*, 2020(8):13–17. doi: 10.1016/S1353-4858(20)30094-5.

Social Care Institute for Excellence (SCIE) (2020) Digital Capabilities for Social Workers. [online] Available at: www.scie.org.uk/social-work/digital-capabilities (accessed 10 January 2022).

Statista, (2020) How Many Mobile Phones in Total Do You and Members of Your Household Use? [online] Available at: www.statista.com/statistics/387184/number-of-mobile-phones-per-household-in-the-uk/ (accessed 3 January 2022).

Stokes, P (2015) Deletion as Second Death: The Moral Status of Digital Remains. *Ethics and Information Technology*, 17: 237–48. https://doi.org/10.1007/s10676-015-9379-4.

Taylor, V (2021) Living Through Covid-19: A Disabled Person's Perspective. In Turner, D (ed) *Social Work and Covid-19: Lessons from Education and Practice* (pp 63–70). St Albans: Critical Publishing.

Taylor-Beswick, A (2019) Examining the Contribution of Social Work Education to the Digital Professionalism of Students for Practice in the Connected Age. PhD thesis. University of Central Lancashire. [online] Available at: https://ethos.bl.uk/OrderDetails.do?uin=uk.bl.ethos.784597 (accessed 10 January 2022).

Taylor-Beswick, A (2021) Social Work Technologies and Covid-19. In Turner, D (ed) *Social Work and Covid-19* (pp 1–7). St Albans: Critical Publishing.

The Carer (2021) Moment in Time-sealed 'Experiences' to Be Opened in 2022. [online] Available at: https://thecareruk.com/moment-in-time-sealed-experiences-to-be-opened-in-2022/ (accessed 10 January 2022).

Turkle, S (2011) *Alone Together.* New York: Basic Books.

Turner, A (2019) Few Social Workers Feel Training Provides 'Digital Readiness' for Practice, Research Finds. *Community Care*, 14 October. [online] Available at: www.communitycare.co.uk/2019/10/14/social-workers-feel-training-provides-digital-readiness-practice-research-finds/ (accessed 3 January 2022).

Turner, D and Price, M (2020) 'Resilient when it comes to death': Exploring the Significance of Bereavement for the Well-being of Social Work Students. *Qualitative Social Work*, 20(5): 1339–55. doi: 10.1177/1473325020967737.

Turner, D (2016) 'Only Connect': Unifying the Social in Social Work and Social Media. *Journal of Social Work Practice*, 30(3): 313–27.

Watling, S (2011) Digital Exclusion: Coming Out from Behind Closed Doors. *Disability and Society*, 26(4): 491–5. doi: 10.1080/09687599.2011.567802.

Zetino, J and Mendoza, N (2019) Big Data and Its Utility in Social Work: Learning from the Big Data Revolution in Business and Healthcare. *Social Work in Public Health*, 34(5): 409–17. doi: 10.1080/19371918.2019.1614508.

Part 2 | Perspectives from Practice

Chapter 6 | Educating the future health workforce for the delivery of twenty-first-century care

Henrietta Mbeah-Bankas

Introduction

Educating the future health workforce has received a lot of attention in the UK and globally, partly due to shortages (World Health Organization (WHO), 2016) but also in response to developing qualitatively different health professionals suited to contemporary health service requirements (WHO, 2013), including technological competence (Topol, 2019). Consequently, pre-registration health professions education has evolved significantly over time in response to the ever-changing health needs and demands of the population (McKee et al, 2021), in parallel with and in addition to the proliferation of innovative technologies. Changes in the selection processes for education for health professionals and in the way they are educated have also been highlighted, with emphasis on the role of technologies in pedagogical approaches to training and development (WHO, 2013; Topol, 2019). This technological emphasis has been further intensified by the Covid-19 pandemic and the rapid shift from face-to-face education to online learning. There has been anecdotal evidence of benefits related to the use of digital and innovative technologies (Warren, 2021; Bramer, 2020; Barber, 2021); however, a preference for a balance between online and face-to-face learning opportunities has also been stressed (Bramer, 2020), resulting in a surge of interest in blended learning approaches to health professions education.

Sustaining the accelerated changes and interest achieved through the Covid-19 pandemic requires a concerted effort by many individuals and organisations responsible for the education of the health workforce. Educators, health profession leaders, regulators and professional bodies have not yet fully embraced the use of current and emerging innovative technologies in educating and training the health workforce, largely due to limited evidence on outcomes (Nursing and Midwifery Council (NMC), 2021). Lack of investment in technology and faculty development are also areas that need to be addressed to fully realise the benefits of blended learning approaches.

Traditionally, health profession educators utilise various approaches to deliver theoretical and practical learning, including digital and online tools, simulation, and immersive technologies; however, their ability to fully utilise these approaches in pre-registration and undergraduate courses is limited by regulatory and other constraints. Individual regulatory bodies have standards guiding expected length, content and outcomes for their specific professions. These can be prescriptive in some professions – from the number of learning hours to be completed for theory and practice, to how many of those learning hours can be achieved using simulation and other innovative technologies (NMC, 2018). Outcome-based regulatory standards should give providers autonomy over the use of technology; however, in some instances, varied restrictions still exist from individual professional bodies like the Health and Care Professions Council (HCPC, 2017) or exceptions from the regulator, the General Medical Council (GMC, 2018). Other limiting factors to the use of simulation and immersive technologies are around the lack of clear definitions of what they are, the quality and consistent provision across all institutions to reduce significant disparity in learning experience for health profession learners.

This chapter will explore how health education provision, particularly pre-registration and undergraduate courses, has evolved during the Covid-19 pandemic, including identifying implications for the future to ensure a health workforce that is adaptable and fit for the delivery of contemporary care. This chapter will also review the benefits of such approaches and contextual factors that facilitate and limit their use.

(Re-)introducing the blended learning approach

The use of blended learning approaches in the education of health professionals is not novel, with evidence of varied use and benefits across post-registration health programmes. However, full integration and use of these approaches in pre-registration and undergraduate health professions education prior to Covid-19 was limited (Health Education England, 2019). Prior to the Covid-19 pandemic, Health Education England (HEE) had started to explore how blended learning approaches could be utilised to promote alternative routes into the nursing profession as part of its mandate (DHSC, 2019). While this was initially met with some resistance, it soon became apparent that the appropriateness of educational curricula and workforce strategies must be reviewed regularly to respond rapidly to education and workforce developments and prevent slow uptake and the dispersion of technological skills (Topol, 2019; Anderson et al, 2021). Additionally, the Covid-19 pandemic highlighted the critical need for such approaches.

Blended learning, also referred to as hybrid learning, is defined as a method of teaching that integrates technology and digital media with traditional instructor-led classroom activities, giving learners more flexibility to customise their learning experiences (Panopto, 2019). For health professions education, practice learning is a key component and the balance of in-person delivery and delivery in a digital environment can vary widely, with regulatory and professional standards requirements to determine how much practice learning can occur in a digital environment. Blended learning has shown benefits such as increased student motivation, personalisation, performance, accessibility and convenience (Bramer, 2020; Lu et al, 2018) when compared with fully face-to-face or online learning (WHO, 2013).

There has clearly been a significant shift in the delivery of health professions education with a demand for digital and online learning, largely accelerated by the Covid-19 pandemic, but the focus must not be on different modalities of presenting information but on what learners learn with innovations in the new environment (Benner, 2000). Equally there are some challenges that need to be addressed to realise the full benefits. These include learners', educators' and technological challenges, a change in culture and resource availability (Barber, 2021).

Learning from the introduction of blended learning to health professional education

Case study

Health Education England (HEE) is responsible for ensuring the education and training of the right numbers of the health workforce with the right skills and behaviours in England. HEE started to commission several universities to deliver fully integrated pre-registration blended learning nursing degree programmes just before the Covid-19 pandemic and has since commissioned others. The commissioned programmes have successfully recruited a diverse student population and have utilised a range of innovative and immersive technologies for theoretical and practical learning. These programmes have challenged the status quo, receiving major modification approval from the professional regulator, an indication of opportunities available to educators to utilise different approaches in educating the future health workforce. Despite the relatively short period of time that this provision has been available, there is emerging evidence that it has the potential to influence the overall delivery of health professional education programmes in the future.

Learners

Healthcare learners are currently recruited on to their courses through their academic achievements and a range of (personally held) principles aligned with NHS values. For a successful blended learning experience, education providers need to ensure that prospective learners have the personal characteristics and an appropriate level of digital literacy to benefit, and providers also need to find ways of providing these additional skills to learners if they do not possess them already (Pusa et al, 2019; Topol, 2019). The emerging evidence from the commissioned programmes also shows that learners who would not previously have explored health profession careers are accessing blended learning courses because of the flexibility offered. Despite the identified benefits and requirements for learners, there are potential challenges that need to be addressed, including access to the right technology, connectivity and student preparedness to fully engage with the blended learning approach (Barber, 2021).

Inclusion and widening participation

While technology can provide opportunities for learners to engage fully in their education online – especially learners who would not typically engage in classroom settings (Barber, 2021) – it has the potential to widen inequalities through digital exclusion for those learners who do not have access to the right technology, for example, equipment capable of running a range of learning software, or suitable learning environments such as quiet space in their home. There are opportunities for education providers to address these issues by providing learners with bursaries for equipment or access to equipped learning centres. Further to this, participation in learning can be observed as, unlike previously in the classroom, many learning packages and software provide analytical functions that can provide data on student engagement. This is important in helping to identify those who may not be participating fully, and ensuring that the right interventions are delivered at the earliest opportunity.

Educators

The professional development of health profession educators is critical to ensure effective educational outcomes from the use of blended learning approaches (Benner and Benner, 2020). This is necessary because of challenges associated with changes to curricula and methods of delivery (Topol, 2019). During the Covid-19 pandemic, there was rapid movement of courses online with technology being bolted on to replicate in-person provision, which meant that the use of these technologies was not driven by appropriate learning outcomes (Barber, 2021). The movement of courses to online platforms reduced the level of disruption to the education of the critically needed health workforce, but it also highlighted challenges for educators. For example, at the start of the first lockdown, nearly half (47 per cent) of educators in higher education did not have experience of digital teaching and learning (Barber, 2021).

Alongside developing educators' skills in digital teaching and learning approaches, the expertise of learning, instructional and educational design technologists is invaluable in helping educators to (re)create teaching and learning materials that are capable of providing essential 'soft' elements of learning, such as curiosity, emotion, authenticity, sociality and failure (Eyler, 2018). It is therefore important that educators develop skills in delivering online and digital education, facilitating simulated practice and the use of immersive technologies, and where this is not available, health faculties should consider using inter-faculty expertise. Establishing academic educators' (or faculty members') skills seems to be limited to higher education institutions with very little attention given to developing their practice learning equivalents (or clinical faculty members), which is central to required experiential learning that health professional education requires. The role of a facilitator is crucial to the success of many experiential learning processes, and undoubtedly to the development of a growth mindset model when using simulation (Warren, 2021).

Technologies

While there has been a proliferation of innovative and immersive technologies in health professions education, there has also been limited research on how technologies augment intended learning outcomes (Logeswaran et al, 2021). Although there are ongoing arguments about limited robust evidence in relation to the beneficial use of innovative and emerging technologies in health professions education, there are reported benefits when used in a learner-centred manner that focuses on learning objectives and reviews the best methods of achieving intended learning outcomes (Logeswaran et al, 2021). These benefits include low attrition rates, improved retention and increased student satisfaction (Garrison and Kanuka, 2004). Technologies allow essential learning from uncertain, fast-moving, unpredictable situations such as the care of Covid-19 patients and other complex healthcare conditions to be captured for education (Fins, 2021).

Achieving effective educational outcomes, however, is based on a combination of factors such as the approach to the design and quality of teaching, and not only how it is delivered (Barber, 2021). The ability to collect data about varied learning activities, regardless of the tools or methods used to deliver them, enables decision-making by and for individual learners, educators and organisations (Topol, 2019). With widening access as one of the fundamental underlying principles for the use of blended learning approaches in health profession education, it is key to ensure individuals from low participation areas have access to the technology, connectivity and space for their learning (Barber, 2021). Skills and expertise required to purchase the right technology is critical to ensuring fit for purpose technological resources are available for learners and educators.

Cultural change

Blended learning health professions education courses promise exciting developments including simulation, augmented and virtual reality, and newer ways of monitoring engagement through data analytics. Developing these opportunities needs collaboration between higher education providers and technology companies, meaningful consultation with staff and learners and a culture that is open to change (Barber, 2021). There has been a shift in perception of the value that blended learning offers but there is still a belief that it provides a 'second-rate education' and is of lower quality than in-person, traditional education. A disruption to traditionally held cultural conceptions of health professions education (eg, exclusive 'by the bedside' learning), particularly in practice learning settings, will be important to sustain blended learning approaches as interest for learners and progress for educators and policy makers.

Ethical considerations

Consideration of the ethical dilemmas and challenges of providing online health professions education is integral to providing an inclusive and safe blended learning experience. The range of ethical considerations needs to be understood through various perspectives, including that of the learner, the educator, the technology being used and interface(s) between all three. Ethical considerations, largely identified and managed by educators, will be key to ensuring that learning technology is not discriminatory, ensures confidentiality and enables learners to act responsibly. Further noteworthy ethical considerations include among others:

> » the blurring of boundaries between educators and learners in relation to communication, privacy and diversity as, traditionally, disadvantaged groups in education systems have similar difficulties in the online context (Anderson and Simpson, 2007; Aldosemani, 2020);

» equality of access for diverse groups of learners (including those with additional learning needs);

» the learners' freedom and blurring the lines between students' and instructors' ethical rights (Aldosemani, 2020; Lin, 2007);

» the use of copyright protected materials.

Conclusion

Health professions education is complex due to the various components required in developing competence (professional, regulatory, theoretical and clinical). Major reform is most likely required throughout the health professions education system to address the rapidly changing needs of patients and the public who use health services (Anderson et al, 2021). Advances in educational technologies have resulted in continuous exploration and use of various approaches to educating the future health workforce(s), including distance, online and blended learning. While the use of innovative and emerging technologies is advocated in the education of health professionals, the drive for its use must be purposeful, complementary and not simply to replace the real-life or immersive clinical experience that practice learning offers. Real-life clinical experience is crucial for developing skilled performance and forming notions of good practice (Kardong-Edgren, 2020), as well as developing expertise and mastery in practice (Dreyfus and Taylor, 2015). It is very unlikely that technologies in the near future will come close to providing the same level of clinical experience to learners as real-life practice.

The Covid-19 pandemic has highlighted the need for changes in health professions education as well as providing significant opportunities to accelerate this change. This chapter has begun to explore the necessary use and implementation of blended learning from a variety of angles. The pandemic particularly identified inadequacies in the digital infrastructure and investment that is required to make blended learning health professions education effective (Barber, 2021) and this will ultimately be a multi-institutional responsibility. While the pandemic has instigated significant learning for all those involved in health professions education, not least our students, there will be a need to continue this learning beyond the pandemic in order to maintain the recently recognised sustainable and resilient features of post-pandemic education.

Reflective questions

» How can the use of technologies and blended learning approaches in health professions education be sustained after the Covid-19 pandemic?

» What can be done to ensure the inclusivity of learners and educators when using current and emerging technologies in delivery of health professions education?

» What mechanisms can be used to capture the teaching and learning experience robustly to influence future development and delivery of health professions education?

References

Aldosemani, T I (2020) Towards Ethically Responsive Online Education: Variables and Strategies from Educators' Perspective. *Journal of Education and Learning*, 9(1): 79–86.

Anderson, B and Simpson, M (2007) Ethical Issues in Online Education. *Open Learning: The Journal of Open and Distance Learning*, 22(2): 129–38.

Anderson, M et al (2021) Securing a Sustainable and Fit-for-Purpose UK Health and Care Workforce. *The Lancet*, 397: 1992–2011.

Barber, M (2021) *Gravity Assist: Propelling Higher Education Toward a Brighter Future. Digital Teaching and Learning Review*. London: Office for Students.

Benner, P (2000) Finding Teaching-Learning Opportunities in the Current Crisis of COVID-19 and the Demand for Online Nursing Education. [online] Available at: www.educatingnurses.com/finding-teaching-learning-opportunities-in-the-current-crisis-of-covid-19-and-the-demand-for-online-nursing-education/ (accessed 11 January 2022).

Benner, P and Benner, J (2020) Designing Online Nursing Education Based Upon Learning Science and High Impact Learning Strategies. [online] Available at: www.educatingnurses.com/designing-online-nursing-education-based-upon-learning-science-and-high-impact-learning-strategies/ (accessed 11 January 2022).

Bramer, C (2020) Preregistration Adult Nursing Students' Experiences of Online Learning: A Qualitative Study. *British Journal of Nursing*, 29(12): 677–83.

Department of Health and Social Care (DHSC) (2019) The Department of Health and Social Care Mandate to Health Education England: April 2019 to March 2020. [online] Available at: https://assets.publishing.service.gov.uk/government/uploads/system/uploads/attachment_data/file/815411/hee-mandate-2019-to-2020.pdf (accessed 11 January 2022).

Dreyfus, H L and Taylor, C (2015) *Retrieving Realism*. Cambridge, MA: Harvard University Press.

Eyler, J R (2018) *How Humans Learn: The Science and Stories Behind Effective College Teaching*. Morgantown, WV: West Virginia University Press.

Fins, J (2021) COVID-19 Through Time. *Issues in Science and Technology*, 37(3): 73–8.

Garrison, D and Kanuka, H (2004) Blended Learning: Uncovering its Transformative Potential in Higher Education. *The Internet and Higher Education*, 7(2): 95–105.

General Medical Council (GMC) (2018) Outcomes for Graduates. [online] Available at: www.gmc-uk.org/-/media/documents/outcomes-for-graduates-2020_pdf-84622587.pdf?la=en&hash=35E569DEB208E71D666BA91CE58E5337CD569945 (accessed 11 January 2022).

Health and Care Professions Council (HCPC) (2017) *Standards of Education and Training.* [online] Available at: www.hcpc-uk.org/resources/standards/standards-of-education-and-training/ (accessed 11 January 2022).

Health Education England (2019) *General Analysis of the Benefits of Flexible/Distance/Digital/Technology Enhanced Learning: A Literature Review.* [online] Available at: www.hee.nhs.uk/sites/default/files/documents/Literature%20Review%20-%20Benefits%20of%20Flexible%20Technology%20Enhanced%20Learning%20%281%29.pdf (accessed 11 January 2022).

Kardong-Edgren in Benner, P (2020) Finding Teaching-Learning Opportunities in the Current Crisis of COVID-19 and the Demand for Online Nursing Education. [online] Available at: www.educatingnurses.com/finding-teaching-learning-opportunities-in-the-current-crisis-of-covid-19-and-the-demand-for-online-nursing-education/ (accessed 11 January 2022).

Lin, H (2007) The Ethics of Instructional Technology: Issues and Coping Strategies Experienced by Professional Technologists in Design and Training Situations in Higher Education. *Educational Technology Research and Development,* 55(5): 411–37.

Logeswaran, A, Munsch, C, Chong, Y J, Ralph, N and McCrossnan, J (2021) The Role of Extended Reality Technology in Healthcare Education: Towards a Learner-Centred Approach. *Future Healthcare Journal,* 8(1): 79–84.

Lu, O H, Huang, A Y, Huang, J C, Lin, A J, Ogata, H and Yang, S J (2018) Applying Learning Analytics for the Early Prediction of Students' Academic Performance in Blended Learning. *Journal of Educational Technology and Society,* 21: 220–32.

McKee, M, Dunnell, K, Anderson, M et al (2021) The Changing Health Needs of the UK Population. *The Lancet,* 397: 1979–91.

Nursing and Midwifery Council (2018) *Realising Professionalism: Standards for Education and Training. Part 3: Standards for Pre-Registration Nursing Programmes.* [online] Available at: www.nmc.org.uk/globalassets/sitedocuments/standards-of-proficiency/standards-for-pre-registration-nursing-programmes/programme-standards-nursing.pdf (accessed 11 January 2022).

Nursing and Midwifery Council (2021) Research into Pre-registration Programme Requirements. [online] Available at: www.nmc.org.uk/education/programme-of-change-for-education/research-preregistration-programme-requirements/ (accessed 11 November 2021).

Panopto (2019) *Blended Learning Defined.* [online] Available at: www.panopto.com/blog/what-is-blended-learning/#:~:text=Blended%20learning%20(also%20known%20as,to%20customize%20their%20learning%20experiences (accessed 11 January 2022).

Pusa, S, Dorell, Å, Erlingsson, C et al (2019) Nurses' Perceptions About a Web-based Learning Intervention Concerning Supportive Family Conversations in Home Health Care. *Journal of Clinical Nursing,* 28: 1314–26.

Topol, E (2019) *The Topol Review: Preparing the Healthcare Workforce to Deliver the Digital Future.* Health Education England.

Warren, A (2021) Using Online Simulation Experiences to Increase Student Nurses' Confidence. *Nursing Times,* 117(5): 34–7.

World Health Organization (2013) *Transforming and Scaling up Health Professionals' Education and Training.* Geneva: World Health Organization Guidelines.

World Health Organization (2016) *Global Strategy on Human Resources for Health: Workforce 2030.* Geneva: WHO Document Production Services.

Chapter 7

Putting down the laptop and rolling up the sleeves: Mobilising a workforce of medical students to the Covid-19 frontline and its impact on their education

George Keal

Introduction

Along with many other professional healthcare programmes, medical students were not immune from the impact of the Covid-19 pandemic. Education and clinical placements were both grossly affected, leaving the traditional medical student experience unrecognisable. With a desire to contribute to the NHS in some way, many medical students offered their services to the frontline but were met initially with barriers to volunteering. As time moved on throughout the first wave, medical students were called upon to assist and underwent bespoke training to prepare them to help in NHS settings in roles akin to healthcare assistants.

With a background as a registered nurse in emergency departments, I am in my third year of a graduate entry medicine programme in the United Kingdom, a four-year accelerated programme for graduates with health or science-related undergraduate degrees. Studying as a medical student and working as a healthcare professional during the pandemic afforded me a unique perspective on the impact of the Covid-19 pandemic on medical student education and preparation to help on the frontline. From this perspective, this chapter discusses and assesses how medical education was adjusted to suit the needs of students appropriately and safely, before exploring ways medical students were able to help in the pandemic.

How did medical education change in response to Covid-19?

Typical educational experiences of UK medical students involve study at a university campus, combined with bedside learning within hospitals, GP practices and similar clinical environments. Traditionally, programmes consisted of a 'pre-clinical' period of lectures and desktop study, followed by a 'clinical' period in healthcare settings.

However, more contemporary styles of medical school teaching now involve a blended approach, with many medical students gaining experience in clinical practice from their first few weeks of their degree, alongside their classroom-based learning. As highlighted by Rose (2020), the transmissible and virulent nature of the SARS-CoV-19 virus meant not only could medical students become seriously unwell, but they could also act as unknowing vectors (in simple terms, carriers). This would potentiate medical students transmitting Covid-19 between hospital wards and, indeed, back to university campuses. Additionally, the educational needs of medical students could prove an incumbrance to overstretched clinicians on the frontline (Miller et al, 2020). For these reasons, traditional teaching practices for medical students during the pandemic were considered unsafe and unnecessary.

All patient-facing activities for UK medical students were expeditiously suspended, including elective placements and clinical assessments involving patients (Alsafi et al, 2020). These drastic changes were shortly followed by incipient cancellation of all in-person tuition and examinations, gradually bringing medical student education in the UK, and internationally, to a grinding halt (Miller et al, 2020). Final year medical students, due to undertake end of programme exams and competency-based assessments required for qualification, were distinctly affected (Choi et al, 2020). A pressing need to graduate and continue to train future doctors meant programmes could not simply be deferred altogether. Medical school education required transformation overnight.

In response to the closure of campuses, Evans et al (2020) explained educators had to shift as much tuition to online platforms as possible in order for learning to continue. Medical schools switched to online learning as the principal form of education delivery (Evans et al, 2020). The required technology for teaching staff to deliver lectures and teaching materials is readily available, outlines Al Samaree (2020), describing it as an excellent alternative to traditional methods. In the months that followed the initial pandemic rules, some schools began to integrate examinations into their online programmes (Watson et al, 2020). However, while the use of online tuition among schools illustrated a uniform approach, the assessment of medical students varied greatly during the pandemic. Alsafi et al (2020) reported that while some medical students had exams either brought forward or delayed, others had exams cancelled entirely, with some final year medical students awarded medical degrees based on prior attainment and performance.

As a medical student nearing the end of my first year, I was in a largely lecture-based component of my programme when the Covid-19 pandemic rules began. In February 2020, we were cautiously warned by the faculty that a short hiatus in education may be forced due to growing concerns over Covid-19. Within a fortnight, all lectures and seminars had been moved online. Our weekly bedside teaching at Royal Hampshire County Hospital had been suspended, with accompanying clinical theory also being taught online. Likewise, fortnightly Thursday afternoon sessions at GP practices were cancelled, now functioning as online seminars. The efforts of the medical school to modify the course to suit a 'working from home' lifestyle was perceived by many students, including myself, as impressive, resulting in a programme that was functional, yet unrecognisable from a few months before. A working week that once required attending lectures, ward-based teaching, laboratory anatomy sessions and primary care tuition now required not leaving the home office for hours on end, and this was difficult to adapt to.

The loss of clinical teaching was sorely felt, with the absence of applying new theoretical knowledge into practice irreplaceable by distance learning. I distinctly recall sympathising with medical students in their later years, missing out on their concluding months of consolidation before graduating as doctors. With regards to tuition, the initial transference of would-be in-person lectures to complete online delivery was challenging for both academics and students, and early on my personal enthusiasm for these sessions was low. With time, many of my lecturers adapted to online tuition, developing more engaging and interactive methods of teaching to suit the virtual environment. This included ideas such as using polls, games and breakout groups for smaller discussions among peers. I felt this facilitated a more productive learning environment, and the benefit of periodic interactive activities should not be underestimated.

Despite improvement in quality, however, quantity was much harder to abide. A medical degree is content heavy regardless, and studying graduate entry medicine, my programme is already five years condensed into four. I was never able to engage with a full working day of online lectures sat at home, finding them gradually more wearisome and uninspiring. I spent much of summer 2020 catching up on content I was simply unable to absorb from the unrelenting virtual lectures of my second semester.

Concerns about the reconfiguration of medical education to the virtual learning environment were raised by Emanuel (2020), who advised that teaching should not focus on time quotas for learning but rather adopt models based on competence acquisition. Additionally, Wolanskyj-Spinner (2020) was apprehensive, questioning the practicability of training doctors within the realms of maintaining social distancing, calling for methods to simulate virtual patient experiences. However, the use of online methods for medical student tuition were not novel at the turn of the pandemic and research by Pei and Hongbin (2019) suggests misgivings about online medical education are unfounded.

In a systematic review conducted prior to the Covid-19 pandemic, Pei and Hongbin (2019) explored the outcomes in the form of examination results for medical students based on their format of tuition. They compared the results of 16 studies, exploring whether online or offline methods had comparable outcomes. Interestingly, no statistical difference in results was noted between medical students who had learnt predominantly online compared with those who had been predominantly taught in person, suggesting that online learning in medical education did not disadvantage students with regards to exam results. Despite these findings, Pei and Hongbin (2019) recommended schools take an approach combining the two methods of education, citing limitations with online learning such as a lack of interactive knowledge building between students and teachers.

Additional limitations of virtual medical education have also been noted. A cross-sectional study by Dost et al (2020) explored the perceptions of medical students concerning virtual education in the UK during the Covid-19 pandemic. A convenience sampling method elicited 2721 medical students from 39 medical schools in the UK, who were asked to complete a questionnaire regarding their experiences of online learning during the pandemic. Results showed that, overall, participants have not found virtual medical education to be enjoyable or engaging, reporting that they did not find it as effective as in-person tuition. Limitations of online learning perceived by participants included distractions from family members and internet connectivity problems. Some benefits to online medical education were also reported, however, including the ability of students to save money on travel, flexibility and the opportunity to study at their own pace.

Additionally, cross-sectional research by Dost et al (2020) using questionnaires found a somewhat unsurprising 75.99 per cent (n=1842) of participants stated online learning had not replaced their clinical experiences, with 82.17 per cent (n=1986) reporting that they did not believe clinical skills could be learned through this medium. The absence, reduction or delay in clinical teaching was found to heavily impact on final year medical students in a cross-sectional study by Choi et al (2020). In a sample of 440 medical students, when asked about the impact Covid-19 had on their clinical education and its impact on their transition from student to doctor, 59.3 per cent (n=261) felt less prepared, while 22.7 per cent (n=100) felt less confident.

While a prompt switch to virtual learning for medical students in the UK meant that medical education could continue, it appears many medical students feel their tuition cannot continue to be provided virtually in its entirety. Benefits to virtual medical education have been highlighted, and it could be argued that the negative connotations of e-learning from the aforementioned studies were biased by students comparing a solely face-to-face education with a solely virtual education. Currently, there is limited published research that evaluates the efficacy of virtual medical education during the pandemic. Nevertheless, the view that medical education cannot function solely online, requiring in-person clinical tuition, is shared by students and clinicians alike.

In what capacity were medical students able to assist the NHS on the frontline against Covid-19?

Relieved of their academic obligations, UK medical students during the first wave of Covid-19 were left stunned and disorientated. Having spent years of learning to think and behave like doctors, the future members of the medical profession were now being met with bewildering demands to stay at home and out of harm's way. Along with their nursing, paramedic and allied health professional student colleagues, medical students were dismissed from wards, while the NHS prepared for one of the biggest public health emergencies it had ever faced. Baker et al (2020) described the paradoxical role of medical students during the pandemic as existing as both the fundamental future of the medical workforce and yet the non-essential workforce in clinical services.

Ingrained professional commitment combined with a sense of duty left an appetite for serving the national response. In a BMJ opinion article, third year University of Leeds medical student Penelope Sucharitkul (2020) said: *'It may be before my time, but we will eventually be the surgeons, GPs and emergency doctors of the future. I can't stand by and let this pandemic blow over without lifting a finger.'* In an interview with the BMJ, Medical Director Dr Kiran Patel, of University Hospitals Coventry and Warwickshire NHS Trust, described being nearly brought to tears after receiving offers of help from such large quantities of medical students (Mahase, 2020). As Covid-19 placed unprecedented demands on the NHS, however, staffing requirements grew and medical students were eventually called to arms.

Medical schools worked with NHS Trusts to find the most productive ways for their students, at differing stages of study, to join the frontline. As with clinical placements, great variety existed between schools and the opportunities their students were presented with. Kinder and Harvey (2020) report medical students working as healthcare assistants and physicians' assistants (note: *not* physician associates) on wards, supporting the ambulance service as community first responders and working for NHS 111. Medical students also helped with many non-clinical roles, including providing childcare support for NHS staff, assisting shielding members of the community with shopping and collecting prescriptions and supporting Covid-19 symptom screening at GP surgeries (Thomson and Lovegrove, 2020). The Medical Schools Council (2020) issued guidance for students volunteering to help during the pandemic, stressing the importance of not allowing it to interfere with their studies. These concerns were echoed by Gishen et al (2020), advising students not to allow additional responsibilities to jeopardise their readiness to qualify.

Within two weeks of my studies moving online, I found myself working again as a bank emergency nurse in a London emergency department (ED) I had worked at prior to attending medical school. Like many of my student colleagues, I had an undeniable drive to assist in the pandemic. Unlike most, however, I was in the fortunate position that I could be deployed as a healthcare professional immediately. On arrival for my first ED shift, I found the department unrecognisable. Like most EDs across the country, it had been divided into a 'hot' and 'cold' area to prevent cross-contamination by confirmed or suspected Covid-19 patients wherever possible.

While back at work I was deployed almost exclusively to the Resuscitation Room, known as 'Resus'. Wearing claustrophobic level 3 PPE for 12 hours at a time, we were caring for an unrelenting influx of incredibly sick patients. Case after case of suspected Covid-19 patients were rushed into Resus by the London Ambulance Service, many in multiple organ failure and significant hypoxia (extremely low oxygen levels). One particularly busy night shift, our patients had consumed seven full cylinders of oxygen just in transferring from ED to the Intensive Care Unit (ICU) – this was unprecedented even for the most seasoned ED clinicians. To put this in context, that is around 3220 litres; when on a normal shift I would not expect to use more than 400 litres. Working back in my previous role, I vividly recall feeling as though we were practising medicine as clinicians but learning as scientists. The pathophysiology and natural history of Covid-19 was not yet well understood; we were learning on our feet while assessing, using any prior closely-related knowledge that could be helpful.

As pressure began to mount on ICUs across London (and indeed the UK), the NHS Nightingale Hospital London was opened. I volunteered to assist and joined as a registered nurse during the second week of operation. Working under the supervision of intensive care nurses, I assisted in the care of invasively ventilated patients requiring extensive support to survive. This was a steep learning curve and it was exceptionally hard work physically, mentally and emotionally. Working 12 hours a day in a warehouse converted to function as an ICU, I remember overwhelming feelings of pride with my fellow NHS clinicians, compounded with anxiety over how the Nightingale was even needed in the first place – why in years before did previous governments not act on our chronically low population–ICU bed ratio (the total population per the number of intensive care unit beds)? Fortunately for the Covid-19 patients of London, the Nightingale was not required for long as London ICUs had managed to expand their capacity to accommodate greater numbers.

After one month of working at NHS Nightingale London, I returned back to ED. By this time, many of my medical student colleagues had begun working both in the department and on the hospital wards as healthcare assistants following a full induction process and training. Even for experienced healthcare students who had undergone years of training, this training was necessary. Owing to the superfluous nature of early medical student placements, consisting of shadowing ward rounds, observing procedures and consulting with patients, many medical students did not yet possess the ability to practise as part of a healthcare team. When asked about responding to healthcare emergencies, Gouda et al (2019) found that only 4 per cent of medical students felt they possessed the necessary skills and experience to help. O'Byrne, Gavin and McNicholas (2020) call for 'pandemic preparedness' in medical student education. They stress the need to prepare medical students so they are able to respond confidently in future and that until that time, they cannot be expected to provide more than members of the public. This is, of course, fundamental in any 'lessons learnt' from medical student deployment as patient safety is always the main priority in any healthcare setting.

The convoluted task of fashioning hospital-based roles to fit medical students at varying levels of training was not so complex for final year medical students. In March 2020, the General Medical Council made the decision to graduate final year medical students early, earning them provisional registration as foundation doctors. Qualifying months earlier than scheduled, the final year medical students were now able to join the frontline as qualified practitioners. A cross-sectional study by Choi et al (2020) found that, despite feeling unprepared, many of the final year medical students felt confident to help during the pandemic.

Conclusion

The Covid-19 pandemic severely affected medical education in both the UK and internationally. The response from schools to transition in-person delivery to online learning was prompt. This enabled education for students to continue throughout the pandemic, preventing the need to defer students or repeat modules. Online learning, however, was not without its drawbacks. Many students found online delivery taxing and unengaging, despite the added benefit of the flexibility to undertake their learning at their own pace. Given the vocational nature of a medical degree, the absence of clinical practice left a feeling of unpreparedness, disproportionately so for final year medical students. With online learning presenting the benefits of remote delivery, flexible learning and an ability to teach large cohorts of students at a time, it is likely to remain a medium for teaching in medical schools after the pandemic. This would be further supported by the currently available, published evidence that in-person teaching does not produce statistically significantly better results. With student satisfaction and engagement at stake, though, the ratio of online learning to in-person teaching needs to be carefully considered.

Owing to their altruistic nature, many medical students wanted to help but were not immediately able to do so. Though many helped in non-clinical roles within the community, it took time and training before medical students were able to be deployed in the clinical environments they had only recently been dismissed from. Despite extensive training in human physiology and healthcare, medical students were lacking in core skills (as well as confidence and experience) to help immediately in the pandemic, raising questions about whether medical students should be equipped with the skills and training needed to help immediately in a pandemic in the future. With this in mind, the oscillation between maintaining patient safety, ensuring high-quality and timely medical education and medical student deployment must be considered through research-informed, co-produced evidence with patients, medical students, academics, government and professional regulatory bodies.

Reflective questions

» What role could online learning serve in the future of medical student education, factoring in the practicability vs the absence from patient contact?

» Given they form the future of healthcare, should medical students' practical exams and exposure be cancelled in response to a pandemic?

» Should medical schools formally train medical students to fulfil an auxiliary role, ensuring they are always prepared for deployment in the event of a health pandemic?

References

Al Samaraee, A (2020) The Impact of the COVID-19 Pandemic on Medical Education. *British Journal of Hospital Medicine*, 81(7): 1–4. https://doi.org/10.12968/hmed.2020.0191.

Alsafi, Z, Abbas, A-R and Hassan, A (2020) The Coronavirus (COVID-19) Pandemic: Adaptations in Medical Education. *International Journal of Surgery*, 78(1): 64–5.

Baker, D et al (2020) Medical Student Involvement in the COVID-19 Response. *The Lancet*, 395: 1254.

Choi, B, Jegatheeswaran, L, Minocha, A et al (2020) The Impact of the COVID-19 Pandemic on Final Year Medical Students in the United Kingdom: A National Survey. *BMC Medical Education*, 20(206). https://doi.org/10.1186/s12909-020-02117-1.

Dost, S, Hossain, A and Shebab, M (2020) Perceptions of Medical Students Towards Online Teaching During the COVID-19 Pandemic: A National Cross-Sectional Survey of 2721 UK Medical Students. *BMJ Open*, 10: e042378. doi:10.1136/bmjopen-2020-042378.

Emanuel, E (2020) The Inevitable Reimagining of Medical Education. *JAMA*, 323(12): 1127.

Evans, D et al (2020) Going Virtual to Support Anatomy Education: A STOPGAP in the Midst of the Covid-19 Pandemic. *Anatomical Science Education*, 13: 279–83.

Gishen, F, Bennet, S and Gill, D (2020) Covid-19 – The Impact on Our Medical Students Will Be Far-Reaching. BMJ Blog. [online] Available at: https://blogs.bmj.com/bmj/2020/04/03/covid-19-the-impact-on-our-medical-students-will-be-far-reaching/ (accessed 10 January 2022).

Gouda, P, Kirk, A, Sweeny, A et al (2019) Attitudes of Medical Students Toward Volunteering in Emergency Situations. *Disaster Medicine Public Health Preparation*, 14(3): 308–11.

Kinder, F and Harvey, A (2020) Covid-19: The Medical Student Responding to the Pandemic. *BMJ Student*, 369(2160): 1. doi:10.1136/bmj.m2160.

Mahase, E (2020) Covid-19: Medical Students to be Employed by NHS. *BMJ*, 368: m1156.

Medical Schools Council (2020) *Statement of Expectation*. [online] Available at: www.medschools.ac.uk/media/2622/statement-of-expectation-medical-student-volunteers-in-the-nhs.pdf (accessed 1 August 2021).

Miller, D, Pierson, L and Doernberg, S (2020) The Role of Medical Students During the COVID-19 Pandemic. *Annals of Internal Medicine*, 173(2): 145–6. doi:10.7326/M20-1281.

O'Byrne, L, Gavin, B and McNicholas, F (2020) Medical Students and COVID-19: The Need for Pandemic Preparedness. *Journal of Medical Ethics*, 46: 623–6.

Pei, L and Hongbin, W (2019) Does Online Learning Work Better Than Offline Learning in Undergraduate Medical Education? A Systematic Review and Meta-Analysis. *Medical Education Online*, 24: 1666538. doi:10.1080/10872981.2019.1666538.

Rose, S (2020) Medical Student Education in the Time of COVID-19, *JAMA*, 323(21): 2131.

Sucharitkul, P (2020) I'm Torn Between Going Home, and Helping the NHS. BMJ Blogs. [online] Available at: https://blogs.bmj.com/bmj/2020/03/27/covid-19-im-torn-between-going-home-and-helping-the-nhs/ (accessed 11 January 2022).

Thomson, E and Lovegrove, S (2020) 'Let us Help' – Why Senior Medical Students are the Next Step in Battling the COVID-19 Pandemic. *International Journal of Clinical Practice*, 74: e13516. doi: 10.1111/ijcp 13516.

Watson, A, McKinnon, T, Prior, S et al (2020) COVID-19: Time for a Bold New Strategy for Medical Education. *Medical Education Online*, 25: 1764741. doi: 10.1080/10872981.2020.1764741.

Wolanskyj-Spinner, A (2020) COVID-19: The Global Disrupter of Medical Education. [online] Available at: www.ashclinicalnews.org/viewpoints/editors-corner/covid-19-global-disrupter-medical-education/ (accessed 11 January 2022).

Chapter 8

Digitalising the volunteer workforce development to support NHS delivery during Covid-19

Craig Harman

Introduction

St John Ambulance is a modern and dynamic charity, but we are privileged to have a long and diverse heritage underpinning our vital work. We have been providing first aid and first aid training for over 140 years. However, our enduring story goes all the way back to eleventh-century Jerusalem where the first Knight of St John set up a hospital to provide free medical care to sick pilgrims. Since then, we have evolved as an order and as an organisation, devoted to our communities, although our volunteer uniform still proudly displays the eight-pointed cross worn by those first Knights of St John. Many people know St John Ambulance as England's leading first aid charity. We train around 250,000 people in first aid each year and our volunteers provide first aid cover to allow thousands of events to happen safely each year. Fundamentally, this work aims to keep communities safe and save lives, but it also supports the health service – reducing the pressures on resources and supporting people's recovery from injury and illness with outstanding care at the earliest stage. The more direct support to the National Health Service (NHS) that we have always given is less well known.

When the Covid-19 pandemic hit the UK in spring 2020, St John knew we had the skills and capacity to help, and rapidly transformed so we could give more. In some areas, such as ambulance provision, we expanded our already existing capacities, but in other areas, such as in hospitals and in the community, our volunteers took on new roles, transferring the skills they already had into new settings, such as providing clinical care in emergency departments. Our involvement in the vaccine programme has built on this work at an even greater scale, training and developing thousands of new volunteers.

From the feedback we have had, we know that the one million hours of support St John has now given have not just been appreciated by the NHS but have had a substantial positive impact on patients and staff. We have heard that St John people have helped give NHS staff time to take a break or focus on more complex tasks, while volunteers have been able to give extra support to patients that staff have struggled to find time to do, in some instances holding the hand of a patient at the end of their life, for example. At a time of pressure and crisis, this support has made a difference to the care patients have received. On ambulances, in hospitals, in their communities, and in vaccination centres, St John people have shown their adaptability and determination to change lives for the better. We now want to ensure that they can continue to support their communities and the health service and that we build a positive legacy for the nation's resilience from the experience of the pandemic.

Mobilising to support the NHS

As the pandemic took hold in March 2020 St John Ambulance's regular operations suffered a major shock. Lockdown meant the immediate loss of two key platforms of commercial income that support our charitable output:

> » Complete closure of our Workplace First Aid Training programmes – this not only affected St John but also the business organisations around the country which relied on us to train their in-house first aiders. In 2019 we had trained 240,000 through our workplace courses. The closure of our training venues posed challenges to our customers, who had a legal require-ment to regularly refresh in-house first aid skills.

> » Phasing out sporting and other public events at national and community level where St John provided first aid services. In 2019 we had attended 20,000 events.

Furthermore, as one of the country's largest youth organisations, we were concerned about the impact of cancelled meetings on our 11,000 badgers and cadets, aged 7 to 17, as they already struggled with not going to school.

However, as a health and first aid charity and England's national health reserve in times of crisis, St John was ready to respond to the Covid-19 emergency. From early January, St John consulted closely with NHS England, with which we already had a strong relationship. It was agreed that we should ramp up our existing support to the ambulance service, as well as provide vital help to frontline medical staff by sending volunteers into hospital emergency departments and other community settings. Within a day of the global pandemic being declared, St John Ambulance launched its Pandemic National Plan, putting an emergency command and control structure in place to support the NHS and our communities throughout the crisis. By 1 April, all St John operations had been diverted to play a role in the national emergency. Our speed of response was unprecedented. Co-ordinated by logistics volunteers, our fleet of 700 ambulances and support vehicles were grouped into 31 emergency regional ambulance hubs for rapid mobilisation; equipment and other kit was checked, refreshed and relocated to make the vehicles action ready.

Other volunteers stepped up to work alongside healthcare professionals in emergency wards including London Nightingale – a 'first' for St John volunteers in modern times. We worked closely with NHS England and hospital Trusts to define their exact role, skills gaps and training requirements. For speed and accessibility, we needed to blend Covid-safe, face-to-face volunteer training with digital learning for the first time. A new training programme was designed, tested and launched within two weeks, a fraction of the time it would normally take. The first trained St John volunteers went into Lewisham Hospital on March 25 and by May, 1500 volunteers were fully trained and ready for deployment. Due to their training, our volunteers were able to support the wider community throughout the pandemic. Working in partnerships in addition to the NHS, St John has assisted with blood donation sessions, cancer screening clinics, home falls and flu vaccination services, as well as providing medical assistance to the homeless and first aid cover for behind-closed-door sports and other events.

St John is built around human connection. Pre-pandemic we were digitally enabled but thrived on face-to-face interaction for training, for development, for support, for routine communication and for our control and command arrangements. From March 2020, commanders sat in their front rooms to lead the organisation, collaborate with partners and to keep people informed. Our units went online, with chat groups and audio and visual conferencing. Our training became blended; the online elements were key to deliver all but the essential face-to-face training so that we could keep our people safe and slow the spread of the virus.

During the pandemic, we continued to support employers, schools and the wider community by developing a range of online modules in physical and mental health first aid, made available free of charge. Working with the Health and Safety Executive, we also offered web-based interim first aid refresher courses to ensure key workers remained safe even if they were unable to formally revalidate their First Aid at Work qualifications. As restrictions first lifted, we designed a comprehensive online resource to help businesses return to work safely and devised our first blended online and face-to-face workplace training. We hosted three national mental health webinars, allowing us to bring professionals together to share workplace best practice when coming out of lockdown, and for our young people we also took our support online. However, during the pandemic, local volunteer youth leaders' weekly in-person group meetings were replaced by virtual modules combining first aid training with fun new activities to suit the media and keep our badgers and cadets talking to one another during this potentially isolating period.

Recruiting, training and deploying 30,000 new volunteers

It started with a request to support mass vaccination sites with some first aiders. By now, though, St John Ambulance's record of upskilling and deploying our clinically trained volunteers where needed through the pandemic, alongside our training expertise, meant that we were well placed to recruit, train and deploy almost 30,000 new volunteers within the Covid-19 vaccination programme. There were to be three roles:

» **Volunteer Vaccinators**, who are administering the vital vaccines. They received extensive training and assessments, including learning how to recognise and respond to medical emergencies. Healthcare professionals provide clinical supervision at each vaccination site to ensure the safety of all patients and volunteers.

» **Vaccination Care Volunteers**, who meet and greet patients and help them navigate the vaccination centre, as well as giving important information about the vaccine and supporting patients who are anxious. Like the Volunteer Vaccinators, they are trained to recognise and respond to medical emergencies.

» **Volunteer Patient Advocates**, who are taught to recognise and respond to patients' needs, including supporting people with impairments. Patient Advocates work closely with NHS doctors and nurses to make sure that everyone feels at ease throughout the process.

Our team of employees and volunteers brought to the national vaccination programme a mix of clinical, training and operational expertise to achieve what was the charity's largest ever deployment. We collaborated closely with NHS England and other partners to ensure volunteers were equipped with the right skills to support the NHS in delivering the vaccinator programme, aiming to enhance the patient experience and deliver the programme quickly to save as many lives as possible. Recruiting and training such large numbers of volunteers required the support of partners such as the Royal Voluntary Service and a huge backroom operation at St John. The 28,000 online interviews were conducted by a 300-strong welcome team, and hundreds of trainers worked quickly to train thousands of new volunteers each week. It also required us to adopt new agile ways of thinking and working.

While some work was needed to check the capacity of our digital recruitment systems, we knew that we would be able to recruit 30,000 volunteer vaccinators in our existing infrastructure. However, as we had experienced earlier in the pandemic, we simply were not used to delivering training, particularly at this scale, online. We had been much more comfortable in the face-to-face space. Our clinical training team supported by NHS England once again worked to develop brand new volunteer courses. To cut down the training time, the new programme used a blend of independent e-learning, live virtual and face-to-face training – the first time St John Ambulance has taken this approach. The result was an overall reduction in training time by one third. At the start of January 2021, the first 400 volunteers were ready to be deployed; by April, nearly 30,000 were ready to make sure the nation got the vaccines they needed to protect themselves and their loved ones from Covid-19.

Leading people through crisis

Leading people through crisis is the most difficult challenge a leader will face. Not since World War II have St John leaders had to lead people through a prolonged period of crisis, where our people were not just impacted by their roles in St John or by the sad nature of what our volunteers were responding to, but also by their own worlds outside of St John changing, where their typical support systems were disrupted.

During a crisis people need to be directed but led compassionately. They also need to be reassured, but they don't see a place for leaders to be over optimistic; they need to belong and feel part of a network of teams. People like to be led well through change, they have to understand the reason for change and what is the long-term plan; they need to be consulted but also know that their leaders are listening to them, and that they have an opportunity to influence decisions. St John's operating model before the pandemic saw volunteers meeting, often weekly, and face-to-face in local or specialist units. Local units were supported by area, district, regional and national teams with access to 24/7 on call leadership support. As is the case in many health organisations, St John has plans to respond to emergencies and trains people to undertake control and command roles during such emergencies, but these arrangements are less favour-able to some and this can negatively impact volunteer engagement.

The pandemic brought many changes to the way that we operated. All activities which were not patient-facing were stopped. Our young people and those who were clinically vulnerable all found themselves at home. Many of our people had to prioritise family, to home school or look after their loved ones, and of course some felt scared by what was ahead. As we entered the first lockdown two things were clear – we would need to significantly change the way we worked to support each other and the NHS, and we were likely to be leading people through a prolonged crisis period. In addition, we would have to manage this process with many of our first line leaders either required to isolate or be patient-facing, and our traditional face-to-face meetings could not take place. Putting in place our control and command arrangements would prove easy, keeping people engaged with those arrangements would prove to be more difficult. Changing the way we operated would also be much easier than keeping people informed of why things had changed and how to do things now. Lessons were learned along the way.

Virtual units created in Microsoft Teams replaced our traditional unit buildings. Designed to keep people connected digitally, Teams offered us an opportunity to allow people to keep informed, collaborate and chat. In our ambulance service this led to the creation of a virtual unit for each of our local teams, providing opportunities for sharing national updates as well as local, very specific items, like how to get in and out of our ambulance hubs, or the entry procedures for a local hospital Accident and Emergency department. When the vaccine programme came along, we did this again to support new vaccinator units. We have had some great feedback about the virtual units but there are some who had a less enjoyable experience connecting online and who grew to miss human connection. We can't forget about people who find technology more difficult to embrace.

The well-being of our people has always come first but during the pandemic we knew that our people may need more support and would need to access support differently. Our leaders would need to be able to signpost differently and be less reliant on face-to-face cues that people were not okay. During the pandemic we set up a dedicated Well-being Cell, chaired by a director, with representatives from right across our operation. We increased the amount of support available to our people and made sure that people would be able to connect with services online and in confidence. We made sure that our leaders were supported in supporting our people too. In addition to our own Well-being Zone, all St John people have access to the HapiApp: available online or by downloading the app, our volunteers could access a variety of support 24/7.

Of course, leading people though crisis and change, particularly over a sustained period of time, and when Covid has also impacted on our leaders, has been tough. Doing so, while adapting to new ways of working and connecting with people, has led to increased pressure on all our people. One of the downsides to the progress we have made in digital connection is the isolation people feel from the lack of human connection. Physical human connection is important for our well-being and for many this feels more authentic than a digital one, particularly for those who are less familiar with technology. As we start to think about our digital future, we will want to embrace the many benefits that technology can offer without losing site of what has made us St John Ambulance for 140 years – our people – and their need to connect with us in many ways.

Conclusion

We believe it is important now to formally recognise St John Ambulance within the architecture of national resilience, to ensure all relevant organisations that may need the assistance of St John's clinically trained volunteers know they can call on us, and can build this capacity into their emergency procedures, resilience and response planning. Our experience during the pandemic has shown us how we are needed as an auxiliary ambulance service. The 158,000 hours of ambulance support we have provided have demonstrated our capacity and strengthened our relationships with national and local service. During the pandemic, St John Ambulance received more demand for our ambulance services than we could meet, and the capacity required during the emergency surge was more than we could currently sustain in normal times, when these levels are not needed. We want to address this by training and maintaining the skills of greater numbers of emergency ambulance crews, vehicles and equipment, to provide more support to Ambulance Trusts when they need it.

Since the start of the pandemic St John volunteers have supported in hospitals in 38 NHS Trusts, giving 136,000 hours of clinically skilled volunteer support. We have received very positive feedback from NHS staff about how much this assistance can be valued. We have also seen substantial enthusiasm from volunteer vaccinators for volunteering with us in future to support the NHS if we are able to give them the right training. We plan to continue to develop our hospital volunteering offer with volunteers and local and national partners, ensuring there's a space for clinically skilled hospital volunteering in future, wherever it is needed. Our reserve of clinically skilled volunteers would also be able to step forward when needed in other settings, such as future mass vaccination programmes.

While we were not a digitally mature organisation before the pandemic, we have had to embrace digital transformation at a faster pace, not only for our internal processes but to reach out, engage and indeed train people in a way that we have not been used to. We must now reflect on what we have learnt so that we can continue to support volunteers and our patients, and serve our communities in a way which is inviting, easy and mutually beneficial, especially as St John now grows into the future.

Reflective questions

» How do you think the NHS and social care organisations can embrace clinically trained volunteers for patient-facing support roles longer term?

» How do you engage with volunteers who want differing relationships with your organisation – traditional engagement models vs an entirely digital relationship?

» How do we make sure that people don't get 'lost' and remain connected, particularly when they need the support of an organisation or their leadership team the most?

Chapter 9

Practice teaching experiences of preparing redeployed workforces for critical care during the Covid-19 pandemic

Timothy Kuhn

Introduction

SARS-CoV-2 virus, a coronavirus disease, is the most recently identified cause of Severe Acute Respiratory Syndrome (SARS) and was first detected by the World Health Organization (WHO) on 31 December 2019, following a cluster of cases of viral pneumonia in Wuhan, People's Republic of China (WHO, 2021). Following the detection of this new SARS virus, Covid-19 cases spread rapidly, and in March 2020, WHO declared the situation as a pandemic. Nearly two years on, by 26 October 2021, globally there had been over 243 million confirmed cases of Covid-19 and 4.9 million Covid-19 deaths, and in the UK alone, there had been 9.5 million confirmed cases and 145,000 Covid-19 deaths (John Hopkins University and Medicine, 2021). The pandemic had and continues to put critical care services under severe pressure, resulting in the need for expansion of critical care beds (and workforce). Due to the unprecedented volume of critically unwell patients, there has been a correlational demand to rapidly upskill non-critical care clinical workforces in order to help care for these patients. In addition to the training needs of the redeployed clinical workforce, there has also been a need to maintain a level of continuing professional development (CPD) for trained critical care staff on managing and caring for these Covid-19 positive patients.

In 2009/10, the novel Influenza A virus subtype H1N1 (swine flu) caused a similar but not as devastating pandemic to Covid-19 and as a result of this 2009/10 pandemic, pandemic planning began across critical care services. An example of this is the CRITCON, a tool developed to examine critical care capacity at times where there is significant pressure on the system, such as during a major incident, winter flu or pandemics (Intensive Care Society (ICS), 2021). The tool was initially designed by the London and Surrey Critical Care Networks following the swine flu pandemic and was then further developed by the Intensive Care Society during the Covid-19 pandemic, and used to help assess whether patients with Covid-19 would benefit from critical care. Alduraywish, West and Currie (2019) state that critical care nurses provide significant roles in the management of critically unwell patients during a pandemic but face many challenges in being able to provide safe and effective care with limited resources and sophisticated infection control requirements. Alduraywish, West and Currie note that in pandemics, critical care nurses need to have a high degree of relevant knowledge and skills to provide care competently but should also be provided with bespoke pandemic education to maximise this care, especially with conditions that do not have a well-known natural history or treatment trajectory.

This chapter is written from the perspective of an experienced advanced critical care practitioner involved in the development of educating redeployed clinical workforces in critical care in a London NHS Trust and a London higher education institution.

Critical care patients with Covid-19

Initially the biggest challenge of the Covid-19 pandemic was that this SARS variant was new and, in the beginning, little was known as to how patients would present and what additional clinical problems the virus would cause. Subsequently, it became clear that patients admitted to critical care with Covid-19 have posed new challenges for clinical staff as not only does the virus cause respiratory failure due to lung consolidation resulting in reduced oxygenation and ventilation, but the pathogenesis of the virus also causes other clinical complications. Clinical decision-making was often made through clinical presentation, the use and review of extensive electronic health record systems in the critical care setting and clinical experience of the clinician (Kuhn, in press). Early in the pandemic Covid-19 patients were recognised to have exuberant activation of inflammatory and coagulation cascades which causes several additional complications. These complications can be identified through laboratory data which demonstrated lymphocytopenia and significantly elevated markers of organ dysfunction, computed tomography findings which showed pulmonary perfusion abnormalities and coagulation abnormalities. Data published from one critical care unit showed that 38.5 per cent of Covid-19 patients had pulmonary embolism, 100 per cent had pulmonary perfusion defects and 18.2 per cent had a deep vein thrombosis (Patel et al, 2020). In addition to these complications, while some clinical trials have shown a reduction in mortality, hospital length of stay and time on mechanical ventilation, there are no pharmacological treatments that have been found to cure the virus. Despite various actions by government and other authorities the rate of infection continued to escalate throughout the following months until the roll out of vaccinations in late 2020 when a decline in transmission started to occur.

Since the start of the pandemic there have been to date 206 randomised control trials (RCTs) which have evaluated potential drug treatments for Covid-19 (Bartoszko et al,

2021). These RCTs have identified that corticosteroids and interlukin-6 inhibitors may have some benefit when given to patients with severe Covid-19, such as reduction in mechanical ventilation time and reduction in mortality. Currently, other medications such as Janus Kinase inhibitors appear to reduce mortality; however, azithromycin, hydroxychloroquine, lopinavir-ritonavir and interferon-beta have not been shown to have any significant benefits. The complex clinical complications and lack of pharmacological treatments have resulted in an increase in length of stay on critical care for these patients, therefore putting further pressures on staffing and capacity, as well as a poorer trajectory for survival. The reported median length of stay for a Covid-19 patient in England not requiring advanced respiratory support interventions is 12 days (Vekaria et al, 2021).

Critical care staffing and nurse education: the pre-pandemic standards

The *Guidelines for the Provision of Intensive Care Services – GPICS 2* (FICM and ICS, 2019) state that at least 50 per cent of nursing staff should have a post-registration academic qualification in critical care. This standard was significantly diluted during the Covid-19 pandemic due to the rapidly increasing staffing needs within critical care units. New staff in critical care prior to the pandemic would have an observed period of supernumerary time and most units would ask staff to work through the national critical care competencies with an allocated mentor, for example, Step 1 competency assessments. Due to the rapid progression of the pandemic and rate of critical care admissions there was not time to provide a supernumerary period and progress through a competency assessment, therefore this was replaced with rapid training focusing on key tasks for non-critical care staff. This brought significant challenges to the NHS, clinicians and, more pertinently, practice educators in critical care environments.

Developments in the critical care workforce

Over recent years critical care has seen developments in its workforce. In response to gaps in the medical workforce within critical care, the Department of Health (DH) and Skills for Health (2008) published *The National Education and Competence Framework for Advanced Critical Care Practitioners*. Advanced critical care practitioners (ACCPs) are highly trained healthcare professionals who have in-depth critical care knowledge, training and experience. ACCPs work autonomously and undertake a number of tasks including but not limited to undertaking comprehensive clinical assessments of a patient's condition, requesting and performing diagnostic tests and performing invasive interventions.

Despite ACCPs being highly trained and experienced clinicians, Covid-19 was challenging as they were also managing these patients who presented with complex health needs and, due to the volume of patients, ACCPs ended up with more responsibility, making more complex clinical decisions than in pre-pandemic times. An additional challenge for ACCPs was interaction with families. Visiting patients in hospital was restricted early on in the pandemic in an attempt to reduce the spread of infection; this meant that communication with families had to occur via telephone or video call, even in end-of-life situations, which was challenging for all staff including ACCPs and families. ACCPs were also involved in the induction and supervision of redeployed staff which resulted in additional pressures on top of clinical activities. ACCPs often bridge between two specialities (for example, nursing, paramedicine, physiotherapy and medical teams) and therefore can be pulled clinically and non-clinically in a number of different directions, as well as having other commitments such as training, education and audit which were all important roles during the pandemic. A sociological analysis of the experience of healthcare staff working during the first wave of the pandemic highlights some these challenges (Montgomery et al, 2021). The study found that Covid-19 caused staff in critical care to experience a situation of extreme stress, duress and social emergency, which led to shared experiences, involving fear and dread of working in critical care, balanced by a sense of duty and vocation. Montgomery et al (2021) also identified that caring for patients and families involved changes to usual ways of working and there was a lack of evidence for treating Covid-19. So, despite these recent advancements in critical care workforce, the workforce was still under significant and unprecedented pressure and the time required to upskill and train new workforces is lengthy. For example, in order for a layperson to become an ACCP, they would have to undertake a three-year undergraduate degree in a health profession, have several years' experience in clinical practice in their graduate profession before then working in critical care for a number of years and then undertaking a two-year ACCP programme. So, while more and more critical care beds can be put in place overnight, manufacturing the workforce takes years.

Creating timely critical care education for registered clinical personnel

The idea of using 'wholesale' blended learning in critical care education was perhaps under-utilised before the Covid-19 pandemic, especially for clinical staff without specific or permanent contracts of employment within a critical care setting. Jansen et al (2021) noted that the Covid-19 pandemic required a time-critical expansion of clinical personnel in intensive and emergency care settings due to the increase of critically unwell patients with suspected or confirmed Covid-19. This chapter now offers two autoethnographic accounts of the author's experiences on two different redeployment courses, including one where he taught content (33n.co.uk learning) and the other which he developed and taught (NHS Trust learning).

Facilitating the virtual and remote learning on the 33n.co.uk

My first experience of formal teaching during the pandemic was the 33n.co.uk course, a remote, online learning multi-professional Covid-19 intensive care unit (ICU) remote learning course for junior doctors (grades foundation year to non-intensive care registrars), nurses, and physiotherapists (any grade) and hospital pharmacists who had been or were being redeployed to critical care. This one-day course was a mixture of pre-recorded lectures, followed by virtual group tutorials led by experienced critical care practitioners. I facilitated virtual tutorials quite a few times over the period of six months. During the pre-recorded lectures and virtual group tutorials, learners gained insight into the basics of critical care and caring for Covid-19 patients. NHS Trusts paid for their staff to attend this course. There was no summative assessment; however, students were asked questions during the tutorials to 'assess' their knowledge gained from the pre-recorded lectures through case scenarios. At the end of the course, students were sent a certificate of attendance.

My experiences of teaching the 33n.co.uk course

The Covid-19 ICU remote-learning course format had its challenges as it relied on learners being able to login successfully and use the virtual learning environment, as well as being reliant on adequate sound and video quality from their homes. The university providing the course did not supply the electronic devices for candidates, so it was down to the individual to ensure they had the compatible equipment. Although delivering the course remotely meant that a large number of people could access the content, it took away the traditional face-to-face element of teaching that I am very accustomed to when teaching critical care to new staff (often by the bed side). Frustratingly for learners and myself, the camera function often had to be switched off in order to maintain connection speeds, which meant that the tutor could not see the learners' facial expressions and thereby gain nonverbal feedback – something I often relied upon in face-to-face critical care teaching.

The tutors also had to adapt to this purely online delivery of teaching and some of the critical care topics were more challenging to explain to novice critical care learners online compared with traditional teaching methods. For example, where I could traditionally draw an anatomical or physiological diagram to demonstrate critical care complexity at the same time as explaining a point, this diagram had to be computerised and formatted to a PowerPoint slide which was 'static' in explaining online, without the more usual 'journey' I could take learners through to check understanding.

Nonetheless, I enjoyed teaching the course, as it felt like students were benefiting from both the recorded lectures and the virtual tutorials. From the verbal feedback received from learners on the 33n.co.uk course, they appeared to be less apprehensive about working in critical care having completed it. This feedback is also supported by a study related to this Covid-19 ICU remote-learning course which examined the pre- and post-course questionnaires which showed that learners' confidence increased from 2.7 out of 5 (pre-course) to 3.9 out of 5 (post-course) (Camilleri et al, 2020).

NHS Trust rapid face-to-face learning

My second experience of Covid-19 ICU learning was an in-person course run by the NHS Trust where I currently work. Three workshops were developed in order to rapidly teach redeployed staff skills that they might be asked to undertake when redeployed to critical care. These workshops included face-to-face teaching stations focused in the main on cardiac arrest management in the Covid-19 patient; intra-hospital transfer of the patient with Covid-19 and endotracheal intubation. Each station took approximately 30 minutes to run. The idea behind the stations was that when learners use these newly acquired skills in practice, they would continue to receive on-the-job training but with other skilled practitioners also in attendance. Over a three-week period, approximately 300 staff were trained. This course was to provide an introduction and awareness of the key tasks that redeployed staff might need to assist other skilled practitioners, and therefore there was no pre-course work or end of course formal assessment, but learners were observed undertaking skills to a tutor's satisfaction as well as asked questions by the tutor during each station. No certificates were given.

My experiences of the NHS Trust rapid learning

Although it was enjoyable to teach and pass on skills to redeployed staff, this course was challenging. The course was taught at the very start of the pandemic and so there were many knowledge challenges. Much of the Covid-19 trajectory was unknown at this time – for example, how many patients would need critical care, or how patients would present clinically and what workforce challenges would occur. The teaching staff had to rapidly learn new critical care protocols that had been developed in order to reduce the risk of spreading aerosols, which was a big concern at the time, so teaching this at the same time was also challenging. An example of this was during the transfer of the critical care patient, where an additional member of staff was used as a 'Covid officer' to ensure staff involved in the patient's care were not coming into contact with objects in the environment such as doors and walls. These changes were outlined in protocols and diagrams; however, tutors had to quickly learn these changes in order to teach and answer questions. Challenges also arose when senior clinicians attending the training disagreed with some of the national guidance at the time. Tutors had to emphasise that much of the guidance being disseminated was not Trust specific but was guidance from national bodies.

Most questions from the learners focused on the procedures themselves as opposed to the Covid-19 specific alterations, as most learners were not from a critical care background. Learners had a general anxiety of the pandemic itself, exacerbated by concerns as to what would be expected of them within the critical care setting. It was emphasised during the training that the purpose of the rapid learning was to give them an insight into some common situations they may be faced with and to equip them with the knowledge of what each procedure entailed. The purpose of the training was not to 'sign them off' as competent and did not replace any existing courses for the procedures taught. Training numbers for each session were limited due to social distancing requirements so the sessions were run back-to-back in order to capture as many people as possible. Staff were also encouraged to read the protocols that had been created which were available on the Trust intranet.

The course feedback was obtained verbally and was generally positive, although some learners stated that they wanted to see the procedures happen outside of the simulated environment. At points during the training, feedback on how a protocol could be improved was obtained and then if appropriate adapted overnight ready to teach the next day.

Conclusion

Being involved in these two courses was enjoyable as it felt like knowledge could be passed on, and redeployed staff received some reassurance about what they might be exposed to; however, each course had its own challenges. There were clinical challenges based on the fact that at the beginning little was known about the virus and how extensively it would affect patients. We could only teach based on learning from other countries' experiences and assumptions of how things would pan out. There were also challenges regarding the wide variety of staff that attended both these learning courses – both courses were open to everyone, therefore teachers had to adapt their teaching styles to ensure that the aims and objectives of the course were met for everyone attending. There was also the challenge of having to teach concepts virtually which would normally be taught face-to-face and creating teaching sessions and electronic protocols rapidly.

Note: The content relating to clinical knowledge of Covid-19 in this chapter was correct at the time of authorship in the summer of 2021.

References

Alduraywish, T, West, S and Currie, J (2019) Investigation of the Pandemic Preparedness Education of Critical Care Nurses. *LIFE: International Journal of Health and Life-Sciences*, 5(1): 40–61. https://doi.org/10.20319/lijhls.2019.51.4061.

Bartoszko, J J, Siemieniuk, R A C, Kum, E et al (2021) Prophylaxis Against Covid-19: Living Systematic Review and Network Meta-analysis. *British Medical Journal*, 373: n949.

Camilleri, M, Zhang, X, Norris, M et al (2020) Covid-19 ICU Remote Learning Course (CIRLC): Rapid ICU Remote Training for Front-line Health Professionals During the COVID-19 Pandemic in the UK. *Journal of the Intensive Care Society*, 0(0). 1–8. doi/10.1177/1751143720972630.

Department of Health and Skills for Health (2008) *The National Education and Competence Framework for Advanced Critical Care Practitioners.* [online] Available at: https://ficm.ac.uk/sites/ficm/files/docume nts/2021-10/National%20Education%20%26%20Competence%20Framework%20for%20ACCPs.pdf (accessed 20 January 2022).

Faculty of Intensive Care Medicine (FICM) and Intensive Care Society (ICS) (2019) *Guidelines for the Provision of Intensive Care Services* (2nd ed). [online] Available at: www.ficm.ac.uk/standardssafetyguid elinesstandards/guidelines-for-the-provision-of-intensive-care-services (accessed 15 February 2022).

Intensive Care Society (ICS) (2021) CRITCON Levels: What They Are for and How They Are Used. [online] Available at: www.ics.ac.uk/Society/Policy_and_Communications/Articles/CRITCON_levels. aspx?WebsiteKey=17ec9561-e0d6-4569-bb31-8fe654a17620 (accessed 11 January 2022).

Jansen, G, Latka, E, Behrens, F et al (2021) An Interprofessional Blending Learning Concept to Qualify Paramedics and Medical Personnel for Deployment in Intensive Care Units and Emergency Departments During the COVID-19 Pandemic. *Anaesthetist*, 70(1): 13–22.

John Hopkins University and Medicine (2021) Global Map. Coronavirus Resource Center. [online] Available at: https://coronavirus.jhu.edu/map.html (accessed 11 January 2022).

Kuhn, T (in press) Electronic Health Records. In Peate, I and Hill, B (eds) *Fundamentals of Critical Care for Nursing and Healthcare Students*. Wiley-Blackwell.

Montgomery, C M, Humphreys, S, McCulloch, C, Docherty, A B, Sturdy, S and Pattison, N (2021) Critical Care Work During COVID-19: A Qualitative Study of Staff Experiences in the UK. *BMJ Open*, 11: e048124.

Patel, B V, Arachchillage, D J, Ridge, C A et al (2020) Pulmonary Angiopathy in Severe COVID-19: Physiologic, Imaging and Hematologic Observations. *American Journal of Respiratory and Critical Care Medicine*, 202(5): 690–9.

Vekaria, B, Overton, C, Wiśniowski, A et al (2021) Hospital Length of Stay for COVID-19 Patients: Data-driven Methods for Forward Planning. *BMC Infectious Diseases*, 21: 709.

World Health Organization (WHO) (2021) Coronavirus Disease (COVID-19) Pandemic. [online] Available at: www.who.int/emergencies/diseases/novel-coronavirus-2019 (accessed 11 January 2022).

Part 3 | Perspectives on Environments, Creativity and Well-being

Chapter 10

Supporting care homes to be digitally connected

Hilary Woodhead and Natalie Ravenscroft

Context

The restrictions on social contact put in place to slow the spread of Covid-19 had an impact on all our lives but were particularly detrimental for people living in care homes. Social contact is essential in the lives of care home residents. Visits from family members and friends are integral to individual well-being and part of care home life, providing companionship, helping with care delivery, and supporting meaningful activity. When family members and friends are unable to be part of care, the well-being of people who live in care homes is at significant risk.

This chapter explores how the National Activity Providers Association (NAPA) adopted a digital approach and supported care homes to consider tech-based approaches and new ways of working during the Covid-19 pandemic. NAPA is a national charity and membership organisation with 3000 care home members. NAPA supports care services to prioritise well-being through the promotion of activity, arts and engagement. We provide support services that equip activity providers with the essential knowledge, skills and resources required to provide person centred, meaningful connections. During the Covid-19 pandemic our flexible and responsive approach enabled us to adapt our support services to be available digitally.

Introduction

The impact of Covid-19 on care homes was devastating. Deaths from any cause in care homes more than tripled and of all deaths that were registered as Covid-19 related in the UK, at least 40 per cent were accounted for by care home residents. Behind each devastating statistic is a person who lived in a care home, friends, family and care staff who looked after them making sense of their loss.

In March 2020, the government recommended that people aged over 70 years should be particularly stringent in following social distancing measures (Gov.uk, 2019). People living in care homes were unable to see family and friends, informal carers or healthcare professionals due to no visitor policies and it was estimated that between 26 May and 20 June, 97 per cent of care homes were closed to visitors (Public Health

England, 2020). Group activities and communal dining were suspended to reduce the risk of coronavirus transmission, adding to the isolation that people experienced. Over a period of 18 months, care homes experienced an extraordinary period of challenge and change. Applying social distancing in care homes challenged staff in many ways and it became evident that new approaches to supporting well-being were needed.

Background

Although care homes had previously attracted criticism for being slow to adopt technology, the need to remain connected accelerated the uptake, showing that it could be done and at impressive pace and scale. At the forefront was the incredible effort and commitment shown by activity providers rapidly adapting their approaches to ensure resident well-being. The most notable development has been the greater use of digital approaches and tech-based activities; this has required an increase in the use of established platforms, more phone and video interactions and a wider use of devices and apps to enable creative engagement. Activity providers were asked to embrace technology and demonstrate their commitment to person centred engagement. To achieve this, they needed support, resources and guidance.

It is fair to say that there were initial barriers to digital connection. NAPA members reported practical challenges such as poor internet connection due to the configuration or design of the built environment and others faced resistance to purchasing equipment or providing training. Direct communication with activity providers on the front line at the start of the pandemic suggested that a number were using their own phones and tablets to enable residents to connect with family and friends. NAPA members reported that with the help of social media, local communities responded with donations of reconditioned electronic devices. Without the support from wider communities some care providers would have struggled to facilitate the social connections needed to maintain an individual's well-being. Later, as the confidence of care homes grew, the government provided an iPad for every care home to enable digital connection.

What we did

Covid-19 was the catalyst for NAPA's own digital transformation. To continue to offer our services we also needed to be creative and innovative in our approach. In March 2020 we made the decision to digitalise all NAPA support services. We suspended face-to-face training, audit and service reviews, conferences and support programmes, and we embarked on a period of transformation. Following consultation with our members, we developed the following digital solutions: e-learning and distance learning courses and qualifications, webinars, an online awards ceremony and conference. We transferred all our hard copy resources to digital download, circulating free activity resources to care homes across the UK, and extended our online presence across social media. This period of digital transformation was only possible due to the support of our members, partners and supporters, with our entire focus on being of use to our care home members at a time of crisis.

In April 2020 NAPA members called on us to publish our position on the importance of activity and engagement during lockdown. Following a period of rapid consultation and in line with government guidelines we published our recommendations; a focus on the need for a whole home approach, one-to-one connection and the identification of key staff members charged with maintaining contact between residents and their loved ones, facilitating digital connection through the means of technology. In tandem we published a series of resources encouraging socially distant activities and providing practical suggestions for one-to-one engagement and creative use of technology (NAPA, 2020b).

As the year progressed and we consulted with the sector it became clear that there was a need for external support and advice for activity providers. In July 2020, with grant support from The Rayne Foundation, we extended the helpline service to include a free phone line, email service and online support group. To date the helpline service has received approximately 2000 contacts. Before the pandemic our responders received calls and emails from care and activity staff, arts practitioners and family members keen to talk through their ideas or their dilemmas. Many of our calls were from lonely activity providers – lone voices attempting to embed well-being into care practice or family members seeking advice on ways to engage a relative. During the pandemic the nature of the calls changed. Approximately 90 per cent of calls to the NAPA helpline became about coronavirus and the impact on activity provision. Approximately 70 per cent were directly related to tech and digital connections and 30 per cent included an element of discourse around tech-based activity. Our helpline responders reported a high level of content acknowledging the essential nature of digital connection, as though it was being recognised for the very first time.

The helpline also received calls for bereavement support and guidance on how to integrate technology into saying goodbye. The way we were all allowed to say goodbye to those we cared for drastically changed as part of the effort to slow the spread of coronavirus. Social distancing advice from the government mandated that funerals could only be attended by a few close family members and friends, meaning many people were unable to say goodbye as they normally would have. The helpline provided practical suggestions to activity teams who reported playing a vital role in coordinating this essential activity in care homes. Acknowledging loss and saying goodbye in care homes is an important part of grieving. We supported members to use technology creatively to say goodbye; examples included contacting crematoriums and requesting live stream funeral services, or using video call apps to help as many people as possible to virtually attend the funeral. NAPA were learning alongside care providers and partner organisations. Expertise from Coop Funeral Care enabled us to develop accessible, practical resources to support care homes to say goodbye to residents and colleagues (NAPA, 2020a).

Inspired by conversations with frontline workers, loss and bereavement specialists and national organisations, we agreed on the need for a collective digital connection to say goodbye. We chose 30 June 2020 as #StarsInMemory Day. Over 30 care organisations joined together in an act of collective meaning making, relieving the 'disenfranchisement' that many bereaved people felt by making grief visible. #StarsInMemory lit up social media as people who wanted to join in on this collective idea put their star up in their window or on show as a public and unified display of grief and loss. Doorways and corridors full of stars and even dancing videos were shared by hundreds of contributors on social media, with the event also shared in the specialist and mainstream media (Care England, 2020). This collective show of the losses encountered during Covid-19 is one way in which the pandemic presents us with an opportunity to highlight the work of care homes and to learn from each other in the sharing of grief. It also highlights the power of social media. We hoped that the idea would spread light and ignite other collective sharing rituals in the future.

Following the success of Stars in Memory, NAPA were approached by Marie Curie who were leading on a national day of reflection to take place on the anniversary of the first lockdown. On 23 March 2021, Marie Curie and hundreds of other organisations including NAPA marked the National Day of Reflection. The nation came together virtually to reflect on our collective loss, support those who had been bereaved and share our hope for a brighter future. Hundreds of organisations, including care homes and millions of people, paused for a minute's silence at midday and many people took to their doorsteps with their own candles, torches and phone lights.

NAPA led a national poetry campaign and published a digital anthology of poetry inviting our members and supporters to write and/or support someone else to write a quatrain (a four-line poem). We encouraged poets to reflect on the pandemic and their experience of lockdown. We were amazed to receive hundreds of digital poems and moved by the impact the process had on many of the contributors.

As the restrictions began to lift, family members and friends began to visit loved ones again and communal activities in small groups were reinstated, we were amazed to see how the arts were being used to help residents express their experience. The NAPA Arts in Care Homes programme announced the theme for its national day and care homes expressed their wish to move forwards by registering to take part.

Most recently NAPA, the National Care Forum (NCF) and Beacon Consultancy came together to create the 'Moment in Time' project. The Covid-19 pandemic was a significant moment in time, which has changed and disrupted people's lives across the globe. This project aimed to capture the range of these experiences for posterity, by creating 'Moment in Time' boxes, which were 'sealed' and will be opened on the same day in 2022. Despite all the talk of a 'return to normal', the pandemic has changed lives in unforgettable ways. This project captured these experiences as a 'moment in time', creating valuable memories and artefacts for sharing in the future. Making and sharing memories in this way has been shown to have positive impacts on well-being, which are much needed after the deprivations of the pandemic. Resources are hosted on a digital platform and downloaded; photographs and videos are shared to enable continued digital connection with the process and with each other as we continue to come to terms with all that has been lost (NAPA, 2021).

Throughout the pandemic NAPA developed many resources in response to issues as they emerged via the helpline. One example of this was in November 2020 when concerns were raised by helpline users regarding singing in care homes. Research showed that there were risks associated with the transfer of Covid-19 through the build-up of aerosol droplets during group singing activities in indoor spaces. The Musical Care Taskforce, co-convened by Music for Dementia and Live Music Now working in partnership with and endorsed by the NCF, NAPA and Care England published *Keeping Singing in Tune with COVID-19 Restrictions* (Musical Care Taskforce, 2020). The resource aimed to help carers and care providers decide whether and how to lead singing and music activities, as well as setting out considerations for planning and risk assessment. The resource highlighted why singing is important, especially during times of crisis. We know that singing plays an important role in care homes and enables conversation and connection, so we shared tools to help staff make informed choices and decisions about whether and how to sing (NAPA, 2020b).

What we learned

The pandemic forced us all to behave differently: to connect digitally we had to embrace the technology that previously baffled us. Care homes responded to the countless challenges they faced with incredible creativity. We have all learnt more about how to use technology, its benefits and its limitations. Technology is now used in a range of ways and more than ever before. Technology will never replace the importance of human connection, but it can support personalised and person-centred engagement and enhance the quality of life of the people who live in care homes. The anonymised examples which follow illustrate the creative ways in which activity providers embraced technology to support people who lived in care homes during the pandemic. They represent a cross section of the work care homes were supporting to embed tech-based activity and engagement during the pandemic.

'John'

Background

John has spent his professional life travelling with the Navy.

John was involved in a road traffic accident and now requires full-time care due to paralysis of his left side.

John identifies as a gay man who is ageing without children – his partner Glen died two years ago and he misses him greatly.

After they retired, John and Glen travelled extensively together.

John says there is no point in living without Glen or the means to travel and feel close to him.

Obstacle

John spends his day sat in his wheelchair; he needs equipment to transfer which causes a challenge when leaving the care home.

John has no family or friends to help him to keep travelling or to live the life he would have chosen before his accident.

The frustration that John feels is resulting in weight loss and lack of motivation.

Support

During a recent online NAPA reflective practice session, the activity provider talked about how best to progress and it was suggested that they try using a recently donated virtual reality system. They agreed the following actions:

» investigate John's life history and travel destinations to build a map of where they could 'visit' with the virtual reality device;

» ask the kitchen team to create a tailored traditional menu of the visiting country for John to enjoy;

» invite volunteers to donate themed memorabilia from places John visited with Glen or is planning to 'visit';

» using Google and YouTube, research languages, music and traditional dress of places John and Glen visited or John is planning to 'visit'.

Result

At the next reflective practice session, the activity provider shared that she had observed an overall improvement in John's well-being. A combined effort from all the departments in the care home had created a person-centred experience. It was also reported that John was talking more about Glen, had put on weight and seemed happier. John had begun sharing and teaching the staff about different countries and cultures he visited. John held his first 'Travel from your chair' session in the home. The virtual reality device has really enabled John to 'turn his chair into a plane' and connect with his memories and life with Glen.

'Derick'

Background

Derick is registered blind and lives with diabetes.

Derick was an independent person who enjoyed writing letters, going to church, taking part in his local quiz group and shopping before his vision became impaired.

Derick has become isolated and feels frustrated.

Obstacle

Derick feels he has lost his independence as he needs support to maintain contact with his friends and write his letters. He does not like to share his personal thoughts with others and feels he should be writing the letters himself.

Derick feels embarrassed to ask for support to complete his hobbies and interests, attending church, quizzes, reading and shopping.

Derick's family are concerned that he is low in mood and worry about his lack of motivation.

Support

The activity provider called the NAPA helpline for advice and discussed how best to progress. The following actions were agreed. The activity provider would:

» share NAPA tech resource with team members;

» support Derick to buy an Alexa and set up an account;

» support Derick to use the device and help him become more independent;

» arrange for the care home to source a booster box for internet speed and fit it into Derick's room;

» brief all staff during handover in how to encourage and support Derick to use his new device.

Result

Derick quickly took to using the new technology with just his voice. Derick found by talking to Alexa he could independently send emails direct to his family and friends once the email addresses had been programmed by the activity provider. Derick also enjoyed independently shopping via the voice shopping list, listening to church services, taking part in quizzes, fitness, news and in the evening listening to Alexa read from the Bible to him. All staff reported they could hear Derick often asking Alexa the time, date or a weather check and enjoy hearing Derick request his morning church service and singing along. Derick's family reported that they had loved receiving Dad's emails, full of news and love.

'Laura'

Background

Laura lives in a care home and has dementia.

Laura has three daughters who would regularly visit Laura for outings, lunch and reminisce with photos or a classic game of drafts.

Obstacle

During the Covid pandemic, Laura and her daughters were unable to see each other and the impact began to take its toll on all involved.

Laura's daughters were keen to find a solution and embraced using Zoom.

Zoom calls caused much distress for Laura, who could not understand how she could see and hear her children on a screen; Laura would often look or walk away.

Laura's daughters became understandably concerned about their mother as they were unable to visit in person.

Staff were concerned as Laura appeared anxious and low in mood.

Support

The activity provider referred to the NAPA resource 'Getting Creative with Tech'. They reflected and talked to Laura's daughters about how best to progress and together they agreed to try the following:

» Laura was offered a space where it was quiet and where she could hear what was being said over the Zoom call.

» A staff member explained the process to Laura before each call, sat with her for the duration and for a few minutes afterwards.

» An ideal time was identified for the Zoom call to take place – 11am, when Laura would be most active and alert to engage.

» The activity provider organised a 'mirror call'. The family would have a draft game set up in front of the camera and Laura would have a draft board set up in front of her. The staff member helped Laura to play with her daughter, moving the counters each time a move was made. This was considered a successful 'visit' and further sessions were planned.

Result

Laura's daughters told the activity provider and care home manager that they felt 'relieved to be able to spend time with their mum and that this was because of the activity provider's well considered use of technology'. They also noted that their mum 'looked well and happy'. Staff reported that Laura displayed signs of relaxation after a Zoom call had taken place. Taking the time to support the session on a one-to-one basis and setting up the 'mirror calls' was a positive and creative use of technology that resulted in meaningful engagement for Laura and her daughters.

Outcomes from a NAPA survey on use of technology

In August 2021 NAPA small survey data confirmed anecdotal evidence provided by helpline callers. In reference to the use of technology in activity provision during an unspecified period prior to the outbreak of Covid-19 in care homes in the UK, the survey found:

» 42 per cent reported 'occasional use of technology';

» 50 per cent reported feeling 'not very confident' at using technology.

In reference to the use of technology in activity provision between March 2020 and July 2021 in care homes in the UK, the survey found:

» 100 per cent reported 'use of technology to facilitate digital connection';

» 100 per cent reported feeling 'confident at using technology';

» 100 per cent reported 'attending online activities with residents';

» 81 per cent reported 'using digital platforms and social media';

» 97 per cent reported 'using NAPA digital resources to inspire activity';

» 53 per cent reported 'receiving no support from their employer on how to use technology';

» 85 per cent requested 'additional tech-based activity support from NAPA'.

Conclusion

There is a need for research in this area. NAPA's small survey data suggests a marked increase in the confidence and use of technology to facilitate digital connection in NAPA member care homes. As we return to in-person interaction NAPA will continue to support care homes to embrace technology beyond the Covid-19 pandemic. We must share the lessons we have learnt and ensure that care homes and activity providers have the skills and resources to further embed technology into activity provision. Each time we use a tech-based approach we have an opportunity to explore new ways to connect with an individual's interests, background, culture and sense of self, allowing us to be inclusive, learn more about the person we support and enable them to remain connected to the people they love and the things that matter to them most.

To find out more about NAPA visit https://napa-activities.co.uk

Call the NAPA helpline free on 0800 1585503.

Reflective questions

» How do you think creative work might support your practice?

» In what ways has the pandemic encouraged your own digital creativity?

» How has the pandemic heightened your awareness of the care home sector?

References

Care England (2020) Stars in Memory. [online] Available at: www.careengland.org.uk/news/stars-memory (accessed 30 November 2021).

Gov.uk (2019) Boris Johnson's first speech as Prime Minister: 24 July. [online] Available at: www.gov.uk/government/speeches/boris-johnsons-first-speech-as-prime-minister-24-july-2019 (accessed 10 January 2022).

Musical Care Taskforce (2020) *Keeping Singing in Tune with COVID-19 Restrictions.* [online] Available at: https://musicfordementia.org.uk/wp-content/uploads/2020/12/Keeping-singing-in-tune-with-COVID-19-restrictions.pdf (accessed 30 November 2021).

NAPA (2020a) *Saying Goodbye: A Resource for Care Homes.* [online] Available at: https://napa-activities.co.uk/saying-goodbye-a-resource-for-care-homes (accessed 30 November 2021).

NAPA (2020b) *Activities in Lockdown.* [online] Available at: https://napa-activities.co.uk/wp-content/uploads/2020/11/NAPA-Lockdown-in-Winter-resource.pdf (accessed 30 November 2021).

NAPA (2021) Moment in Time. [online] Available at: https://napa-activities.co.uk/services/training/a_moment_in_time (accessed 30 November 2021).

Public Health England (2020) COVID-19: Number of Outbreaks in Care Homes – Management Information. [online] Available at: www.gov.uk/government/statistical-data-sets/covid-19-number-of-outbreaks-in-care-homes-management-information (accessed 30 November 2021).

Chapter 11 | Creative social work in a virtual world: A case study on a work-based learning module

Michaela Dunn, Rachel Parry Hughes and Andrew Linton

Introduction

The coronavirus pandemic catapulted our teaching to an online learning environment, changing the interaction between students and educators, forging new, dynamic and flexible approaches in our work-based learning modules for social workers and social care practitioners.

One such module connected the world of art with that of social work, empowering practitioners to embrace and utilise creative approaches to connect with vulnerable children, young people, adults and families in a diverse London local authority.

Our case study will examine how we shifted what was an in-person, interactive module to one where we connected in ways unimagined and unexpected within a virtual environment. We will explore the themes of creativity, connection and the relationship-based nature of social work that continued to shine despite the often impersonal nature of a virtual screen. We will consider the practitioner viewpoint and their contribution to this module, exploring and expanding upon the inherent need for creativity in social work and how this may translate into practice.

New Town Culture

In 2020, we at Goldsmiths were commissioned by the London Borough of Barking and Dagenham (LBBD) to carry out work on the second phase of 'New Town Culture' (NTC), a pioneering programme bringing together the arts and social work through collaboration between LBBD's Children's Social Care department and national and local cultural organisations. The overarching aim of the programme is to explore how artistic and cultural experience can enhance the work of social care practitioners and thus help to support adults and children in need of social care services. The programme has pursued three strategies for achieving this aim. Firstly, it has increased the arts offer to young people and adults using LBBD social care services by running an extensive programme of arts-based clubs and workshops. Secondly, it has sought to make creative activity an integral part of the local authority's systems and processes within its work with residents; for example, it has provided funding for a cultural practitioner to work within LBBD's specialist intervention service for young people. Finally, it has promoted a cultural exchange of ideas and expertise between the arts and social care sectors.

We had already been part of that exchange, working with LBBD on the first phase of the NTC programme (2018–20) and we welcomed the opportunity to continue working with them and cultural partners on the ideas we had developed together. These ideas are set out in our report *The New Town Culture Programme 2018–2020: Art, Creativity and Care* (Hughes et al, 2020). In the second phase of the project, the aim was to share these ideas more widely within LBBD's Children's Social Care department, so that they could be shaped by the social care workforce going forward. We worked with the New Town Culture curatorial team on a number of ways of doing this, including our Interdisciplinary Intervision programme (Hughes et al, 2020) and the initiative which is the focus of this chapter: a Level 7 (master's) module in work-based learning with a focus on 'creative social work'.

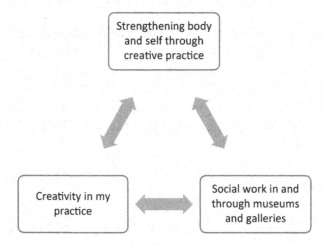

Figure 11.1 Structure of the creative social work module

Figure 11.1 shows the overall structure of the creative social work module: three inter-related areas of learning, with each area of learning being facilitated by a three-member team of social worker, cultural practitioner (artist or curator) and expert by experience (EBE). Each team received a 'brief' for their area of learning (written by Rachel Parry Hughes in collaboration with the NTC curatorial team) which included five suggested learning outcomes. These learning outcomes were derived from existing work within the NTC programme. For example, one of the outcomes for the 'strengthening' area of learning was for students to have the opportunity to reflect on how they experience resilience and resistance in their own bodies and minds. This outcome was inspired by the work of the artist Helen Cammock and LBBD youth offending practitioners, which we at Goldsmiths had observed as part of our research on the first phase of the NTC programme. The learning outcomes in the 'creativity in my practice' area of learning focused on identity and drew on a piece of work by artist Albert Potrony and unaccompanied asylum-seeking young people called 'Make Your Own English' (Hughes, 2020). In all areas of study, a learning outcome was included to encourage students to consider the intersectional impact of race, gender, sexuality, age, socio-economic class and other markers of identity. Crenshaw's (1994) intersectionality is integral to teaching and learning at Goldsmiths, but this was given additional urgency and focus by the death of George Floyd in May 2020, just as we were working on the module design (Reid, 2020). Beyond the constraints of the 'five learning outcomes', the facilitation teams had 'free rein' to develop content, materials and methods of delivery. This kind of freedom is as integral as intersectionality to our shared philosophy of teaching within the social work team at Goldsmiths. We had reason to be glad of this freedom when it became clear that there would be no face-to-face teaching happening in autumn 2020 and our creative social work module would have to go entirely online.

Movement to online platform

The creative social work module was facilitated over three study days during one term. Within this the 'Creativity in My Practice' study day was the second day, divided into two sessions, one focused on identity and the other focused on memories. For the discussion below, the focus will be on this second day. The main facilitators collaboratively involved in both the planning and delivery of the teaching and learning activities were Goldsmiths social work lecturers Michaela Dunn and Andrew Linton, artists and curators Albert Potrony and India Harvey, and members of the Goldsmiths EBE group (individuals with lived experience of social care services). The sessions were jointly planned based on the dedicated brief provided by NTC and these were incorporated into learning outcomes for the sessions. As noted above, the facilitators discussed and agreed that it was important to promote practitioner free thinking and opportunities to be creative within the teaching and learning activities. This was further energised and promoted through connecting different disciplines, approaches and ideas. There was also apprehension in moving what was intended as a face-to-face session to an entirely online platform.

Perhaps most significant in shifting an entire continuing professional development (CPD) module from in person to online was a rethinking of platforms where the cultural and creative exchange could occur and be felt.

Hughes et al (2020, p 8) summarises this need as follows:

The coronavirus pandemic provided a pause to our work and an opportunity to rethink how we would achieve this aim of cultural exchange, and the first few weeks of lockdown acted as a crucible for forging new ideas. We realised that what was needed for the workers was in fact something like what we had seen the artists creating so successfully for young people: a space and form of activity which allowed for an exchange on equal terms and the creation of new narratives of (professional and personal) identity and practices which may transcend existing mindsets and cultures.

Consideration was given as to how best to 'take care' of one another and the space virtually. There was a mindfulness of the pandemic's often described characteristics – leading to isolation, worry, stress and ultimately trauma. Social care practitioners felt the weight of this pressure throughout the pandemic, with at times lingering effects, thus in planning there was even more emphasis on a safe, shared online learning environment to acknowledge, share and offload some of this weight (Bennett et al, 2021). Contemplation was given on how best to translate the dynamic and unique material of the creative social work course to (what may be considered) the impersonal, stale and potentially one-dimensional platform of the virtual classroom: how to enable the learning and teaching to take on characteristics of being trauma-informed, mindful and caring (Carello and Butler, 2015). The shift was in acknowledging the challenges and prioritising at every juncture the need for teaching and learning that is both sensitive and caring. The emphasis became a redistribution of power in the virtual setting, encouraging cultural humility in sessions without expertise positioned in one or two individuals. Rather, a social pedagogical approach was employed, recognising everyone as teachers, not only an acknowledgement but a deep appreciation of the individual, their identity and bringing this appreciation, this humility, into the session to enact and engage curiosity (Bennett et al, 2021). The teaching and learning promoted interaction and conversation, increasing reflective and reflexive discussions. In planning the sessions, the lecturers, artists and EBEs were in turn the visual guides, with the discussions and activities led and directed by practitioners. 'Taking care' was encouraged throughout the session: a check-in at the beginning encouraging a moment of self-care, regular screen time breaks were included throughout and 'breakout rooms' to open up meaningful discussions, modelling for one another a soft space to relate and connect through compassion and care.

The 'Creativity in My Practice' study day focused on why memories matter, the experience of memory in art, 'who do we think we are' and how art and creative practices can be a tool to explore identity and self-narrative in social work practice. The day session provided a space to explore identity narrative, memories, needs and culture, both personally and professionally. The question posed was as social care and social work practitioners, how can we demonstrate anti-oppressive work in our actions and interventions by gaining insight and understanding of our own identity?

Artist Albert Potrony identified the work of two artists – visual artist Abraham Cruzvillegas and performance artist Nick Cave – who each in their own way explore identity through their art. Cave offers the concept of 'a new skin' to transcend how we may typically define or label identity. In social work, this can be related to Burnham's (2012) Social GGRRAAACCEEESSS, an acronym of wider descriptions ascribed to personal identity. Cave suggests that we can transcend the ascribed social identities by creating a new one of our own. Cruzvillegas' work explores identity through that of a 'transparent' one, an identity that is ever evolving and influenced by our experiences. 'Who we are' is constantly being constructed – as a building may be made, our identity is formed of 'building blocks' consisting of people, experiences, memories, objects and connections that contribute to the making of who we are. Potrony transformed the work of Cave and Cruzvillegas into two tangible activities for the practitioners to complete, creating either a new skin (by using material available in the home environment) to transcend ascribed labels and categories of identity or a piece of work (either a collage, video, or audio depiction) that revealed how their identity has been constructed. It was important for the activities to be accessible and transferrable, thus practitioners were encouraged to use what was available in their own space, be that either in the office, or, for most participants, in their home environment. Participants were encouraged to have fun in creating art, using their imagination to explore their own identity. Practitioners had a protected time to create their own artwork, free from the screen, but able to 'check-in' with one another if needed as they were moved into breakout rooms.

Practitioners had the opportunity to safely explore and share aspects of their identity with experimenting in this creative-based activity. Following the activity, practitioners shared with one another the art created, explaining the significance of what they included in the piece, empowering each other with sensitivity and care to be vulnerable, revealing part of their personal selves to one another. This bonding action of sharing self through art fostered respect and empowerment, key mechanisms of relationship-based social work practice (Ruch, Turney and Ward, 2018). By completing the activity, practitioners were able to directly take part in the experiential learning, enabling opportunities of 'ah-ha' moments, promoting not only growth and connection, but also how to translate this learning to practice.

The study day prompted practitioners to explore how this creative approach could relate to social work practice. Particularly with Cave's artistic work, the practitioner is asked to reflect on what aspects of identities are seen or hidden in the interventions. There was reflection on the visibility of service users during the pandemic – impacted by isolation and social distance – and that vulnerable individuals may be without family and social support networks and so in turn may not be seen (Neha, 2021). The activities explored individual identity through sharing diverse backgrounds, experiences and influences, how in turn we may be seen and how we see one another. Practitioners were encouraged to adapt the activities for their own settings with service users and maintain creative links in their practice to uncover aspects of identity that need to be heard or made visible. Key to social work practice is promoting diversity and equality and the creative activities elevated this pursuit in bringing visibility to the individuals' experience, their narrative and their identity.

Practitioner feedback

Evaluation of the module consisted of two methods: feedback sought after sessions via short questionaries and feedback sought during focus groups, which is the source of evaluation reviewed for this discussion. There were two focus groups attended by six practitioners out of a total of 18 who participated in the CPD course. Focus groups were recorded and transcribed. Questions and thus emerging themes from the focus groups related to practitioners' motivation to take part, challenges faced and the overall impact of the course on the individual and their social work practice.

Practitioners were motivated to take part in the creative social work course due to intrigue and interest in the title and subject matter, with the added wish to embrace that potential of working creatively in their practice.

So I wanted to do it, as I really love that title, creative practitioner, I think that's a compliment. And I'd love to have that, to be able to say, I've done this course, you know, and that I was successful. Because I suppose I hope that I am a creative practitioner, and I suppose I like to think that I am.

(Practitioner Two)

Practitioner Three added that not only the title, but widening the scope of resources could impact on how to engage:

I think for me...the course title is very attractive. We need a lot of creativity in our work, we work with the different families, different children, some are willing to work with us straightaway, some not willing... so we always need a creative approach, we have to think outside the box all the time, with the different challenges that we come across in our professional practice. So something... to be equipped with more resources, more creativity is quite essential in this job.

Practitioners shared that they felt face-to-face teaching may have provided opportunities to network, for example, going out to lunch with one another and supporting each other with assignment queries. The major benefit of working from home was that of convenience; however, for some, if they were not on an external training course 'outside of the workplace', then there may be expectations to complete work at home. Practitioners openly shared some of the complexity and pressure of their work during the pandemic, not only in all the different roles they needed to fulfil – such as a social worker, manager and/or support worker – but also the increased workload and associated stresses relating to a global pandemic linked to insecurity, worry and fear.

One practitioner queried *'do we know how to do it?'*, the how as 'well-being' and an additional question *'do we resist looking after ourselves as social care practitioners?'* Practitioners reflected that the course offered a pause to this turmoil and stress of the work day, a literal break to reflect on one's well-being, practice and the creative arts. Moving from the feelings of burnout and emotional drain of the work and self-describing as 'recovering social workers', there was a shared sentiment of being suspended in crisis interventions during the pandemic. However, the learning and teaching within the creative social work module supported and promoted active recovery. Practitioner Five shared the following:

And I feel because the young people that I've been working with, they have struggled a lot through this lockdown. And instead of, you know, because as much we're human at the end of the day, and we don't want to project, whatever, we're feeding onto these kids or whatever, but we're human, you know. But it's actually just made me just sort of breathe and say, right, step back...whatever I can do with that young person and sort of go through and all the little things that I've been doing to get myself back in line, I've been passing it on to them. So that's what's been the, I would say, it's been absolutely great with this course, because it's really sort of brought me back to the ground.

The creative social work course could be used not only as a tool, but as a conduit to that connection and the draw to humanity, promoting active ways for individuals to support one another with open, honest and vulnerable discussions. Practitioner Six shared their recent experience of being moved to a new and unfamiliar team and the benefit of the course on their resilience, well-being and practice:

But it just opened my eyes to what I could do in a different environment when I am working with my clients. So it has given me confidence, even though it is a very unfamiliar area that I've been asked to go and work, to know that I will survive there.

The course further expanded the ability to create safe spaces to foster honest authentic interactions and conversations. Participation in the course generated a sense of belonging to a context in which practitioners could emotionally engage and feel part of something special. This has been evident throughout the teaching of the module and present during the focus groups, with lots of excitement articulated by practitioners keen to return to the materials and learning. There was throughout a shared acknowledgement by both presenters and participants that the arts and creativity is fundamental in people's lives, with a unique impact on practitioner well-being and social care practice.

Reflective questions

» How are you seen by others in your practice?

» Which parts of your identity are evident in your practice?

» How significant is creativity in your practice?

References

Bennett, B, Ross, D and Gates, T G (2021) Creating Spatial, Relational and Cultural Safety in Online Social Work Education During COVID-19. *Social Work Education*. doi: 10.1080/02615479.2021.1924664.

Burnham, J (2012) Developments in the Social GGRRAAACCEEESSS: Visible Invisible and Voiced-Unvoiced. In Krause I (ed) *Culture and Reflexivity in Systemic Psychotherapy: Mutual Perspectives*. London: Karnac.

Carello, J and Butler, L D (2015) Practicing What We Teach: Trauma-Informed Educational Practice. *Journal of Teaching in Social Work*, 35(3): 262–78.

Crenshaw, K (1994) Mapping the Margins: Intersectionality, Identity Politics and Violence Against Women of Color. In Fineman, M A and Mykitiuk, R (eds) *The Public Nature of Private Violence* (pp 93–118). New York: Routledge.

Hughes, R, Steedman, M and Staempfli, A (2020) The New Town Culture Programme: Promoting Cultural Exchange between Artists and Children's Workers. *Youth and Policy*, pp 1–9. [online] Available at: www.youthandpolicy.org/articles/new-town-culture/ (accessed 16 January 2022).

Hughes, R (2020) *The New Town Culture Programme 2018–2020: Art, Creativity and Care*. Interim Report. [online] Available at: https://newtownculture.org/resources/evidence/the-new-town-culture-programme-2018-2020-art-creativity-and-care/ (accessed 6 November 2021).

Neha, S P (2021) Encouraging Multiculturalism in Social Work Education and Practice: Responding to Covid-19 Pandemic. *Social Work Education*. doi: 10.1080/02615479.2021.1887118.

Reid, W (2020) Black Lives Matter: Social Work Must Respond with Action – Not Platitudes. *Community Care*, 6 December. [online] Available at: www.communitycare.co.uk/2020/06/12/black-lives-matter-social-work-must-respond-action-platitudes/ (accessed 10 November 2021).

Ruch, G, Turney, D and Ward, A (2018) *Relationship-Based Social Work: Getting to the Heart of Practice* (2nd edition). Philadelphia: Jessica Kingsley Publishers.

Chapter 12

Mindfulness, social work leadership and Covid-19

Annie Ho

The practice of mindfulness

The practice of mindfulness is becoming increasingly popular and has wide application for a range of personal and professional disciplines. Practising mindfulness could be seen as an antipathy to social work practice, considering the pressures and demands of the job. However, mindfulness techniques can help to slow down reactivity, avoid habitual responses and allow new creative solutions. A mindful social work leader can help to grow mindful practice, improving the well-being of social workers and therefore the well-being of the people we work with. This chapter, written from the perspective of a principal social worker and manager, charts my experiences of applying mindfulness during the Covid-19 pandemic and explores the potential value of mindfulness in bringing in an attitude of curiosity, sensitivity and kindness to social work practice. The move to digitalised solutions in social work has brought about ethical challenges to the profession but, perhaps in other ways, allowed the development of these new ways of working.

Everything was cancelled

26 March 2020 was a memorable World Social Work Day. Six months into my position as principal social worker, I was ready to make a difference. I spent months preparing for a week of talks and activities for our workforce. Lockdown struck and everything was cancelled at short notice. The one in-house event which went ahead was a five steps to mental well-being workshop where my public health colleagues and I offered what we could to a workforce in shock. I quickly changed what I was going to say and managed to put together a short presentation under the banner of the International Federation of Social Workers, remembering our colleagues worldwide as we stood together to advance our common message globally at the start of the pandemic.

The phenomenal speed of change to remote working and Teams meetings allowed us to practise well-being during lockdown, through connecting to nature when we took breaks from our screen. When I asked my social workers whether they had had their daily physical exercise, I asked myself the same question and had to make myself stop and go out for a walk. We publicised resources including apps on mindfulness, sleep, fitness and art and craft. One social worker from Italy shared about converting his outdoor bike to an indoor exercise bike and watching videos of cyclists in the beautiful Italian mountains while on his turbo bike.

Like many managers, I was, however, reticent about supervising my staff on a computer screen. Remote supervision is as foreign to me as remote assessments are for social workers. Domakin (2020) provides a helpful reminder that effective supervision is relational, emotionally literate, reflective and curious regardless of whether you connect virtually or in person. The metaphor of the gearstick is used to help us think about how we can move from fourth gear – working at top speed to get things done, to first gear – where we can listen and attend in supervision.

Social work managers should be aware that supervision always starts with the well-being of the staff we supervise, before we get to the tasks which need to be achieved. While the intention has always been there for me to find time before entering into a supervision physical space, the reality of a busy office doesn't always allow for the necessary preparation. Remote supervision has made it possible for me to be more prepared and more attentive to the individual social worker across the screen. When I get to the first standing agenda item of well-being, I am keenly aware that my staff are working at home, with potential interruptions from children, pets and deliveries. I am aware of the limitations in picking up visual cues remotely and so I need to be sensually attuned and emotionally available in the present moment. I am more mindful of checking in with my staff, allowing more time and space for them to share how Covid is affecting them, both professionally and personally.

We survived the early days of crises, when everything was either cancelled or moved online. In many ways, the pandemic has provided a place for individual and collective humanity to come together. The remote platform has, perhaps unintentionally, offered a virtual place and space for the 'meeting' between the leader, manager or supervisor and the social work practitioner, where humanity and emotions can be more meaningfully acknowledged and explored than in the physical, often harsh, office environment. We now need to move beyond and do more than simply offering online resources and the IT infrastructure to enable our staff to cope. We now need leaders who deeply care and truly inspire our staff to thrive.

Creating a space for reflection

A survey published in March 2019 by *Community Care* (Stevenson, 2019) concluded that hotdesking, often a council-wide policy, negatively impacted on the enjoyment and effectiveness of social workers at work. Aside from the obvious focus on improving remote technology, the *Community Care* research offered suggestions on how to improve the hotdesking experience for social workers, including improving storage options for individual staff in the office and creating a more homelike atmosphere. The ability of social workers to include personal touches in their individual work-space can help their motivation. It is difficult to make an open plan office homely, but small things can make a big difference.

Having been in local authority social work for over 30 years, I remember the old-fashioned building which was my first office, with long corridors and individual team rooms. I was the aspiring social worker who became the senior practitioner and then the team manager, enjoying the space of a room of my own, adjacent to the room of my team. The team culture was built within this reflective space. The manager's door was left open for a large part of the day, but my team respected the time when I had my door shut and needed space on my own. When I returned to this office after my one-year maternity leave, Jane came up to me with her tea trolley and remembered exactly how I took my tea – very strong and no sugar! As a manager, I had no intention of hiding the fact that I'm also a proud mother, so the photos of my children are placed prominently on my desk. Those days are so distant from the open plan office and clean desk policy of the last ten years of my working life. I used to put some personal, senti-mental items in my locker and took them out for placing in my workspace every day, as I needed to be reminded in the course of my busy working day to be mindful and grateful. As time went on, the pressures of work continued to pile on and I couldn't even find the time to think about these special objects, never mind taking them for a tour round the office until I identified and quickly snatched a free desk.

Creating space for reflection should result in a reduction in stress and pressure on social workers and an increase in efficiency. While informal discussion with managers and colleagues across the desks and by the water cooler or the printer in the office is no longer a regular occurrence, sharing and checking out can take place instantly over Teams chat and video conferencing. Remote working from home, where the home environment allows, can create the time and capacity for social workers to be more reflective in their work.

It is more important to me to be a mindful, kind and curious leader, even though I rec-ognise I need to keep my manager's hat on. If I lead well, I believe I will manage well. I am beginning to learn to use remote platforms to my advantage to get to know staff holistically. When I asked questions about my staff well-being in the past, I allowed them to bring in their family and whatever parts of their personal life they are com-fortable with sharing and they feel are having an impact on their work. When I show genuine interest in my staff well-being now, I have no choice but to accept that their work and home have come together and one is inevitably impacting on the other. 'Meeting' on the remote platform over the course of the pandemic has an impact in some way by equalising the relationship between the one who leads and the one who is being led. There is less power imbalance and less divide, due to the commonality of experience of trauma and suffering from Covid. 'Cultural humility' helps us avoid 'othering' the other person – under the threat of the pandemic, the 'them' and 'us' division does not exist (Treisman, 2018).

Grief and loss

In March 2020, *Community Care* reported that '*A social worker at a London borough has died after being infected with coronavirus, the local authority's leader said today*' (Turner, 2020). Imagine, on top of the whole nation's unpreparedness for the sudden arrival of the pandemic, the shock experienced by all council staff of this particular London borough – the borough where I work. Imagine too, the grief and fear of our social workers as *Community Care*'s headline news on coronavirus was specifically focused on one of our colleagues. On the same day, our leader announced that one employee of our street cleaning team also lost their life to Covid. Then the figures started going up – 10 social workers (Samuel, 2020a), 21 social workers (Samuel, 2020b), 36 social workers (Carter, 2021), and so it continues. Social workers persist in their everyday work to uphold value-based and rights-based social work, while taking on this additional title as 'key workers' in the fight against the pandemic, hearing the daily message on their TV screen and social media that social care is being 'neglected' during the pandemic.

How do we meaningfully pay tribute to these colleagues and the service users we lost during the pandemic? The period between March and December 2020 was relentless – there was no time for mindfulness or reflection; it was purely and solidly getting my head down. All my booked leave was cancelled and I was happy to cover Christmas so that my staff could have a break.

When January 2021 started with the news of the sudden death of a social worker I 'met' remotely a few weeks previously for discussion on a complex case, I stopped. I finally stopped to grieve about three personal friends I lost in the last year, which I never 'brought to work'. I also stopped to listen to the personal stories of so many staff members – loss of family, friends, colleagues and service users – and decided I needed to put the brakes on and encourage everyone to do the same, before we could move forwards together again. We had an online grief and bereavement session together where, for the first time, I brought along my three dead friends and paid respect to them, as managers and social workers remembered their colleagues and loved ones.

'Every interaction is viewed as an intervention, as an opportunity for change, as a possible sparkle and turnaround moment, and as an opportunity for the values to be modelled and embodied' (Treisman, 2018). As a mindful leader, I believe that every interaction with our staff and every interaction with people we work with provides that unique opportunity. It is incumbent on us as leaders to model and embody the values and commitment we expect from our staff. I can put my finger on those precise 'sparkle' and 'turnaround' moments on the long road we have been travelling together since the first lockdown. The 'sparkle' provided by the online grief and bereavement session enabled me to pick myself up and get back on the road. I believe it did something special in different ways for different people attending the session.

Kindness and curiosity

Mindfulness must come with kindness and curiosity. Kindness is a word which appeared to have gone out of fashion, to perhaps reappear during the global pandemic, as we have been witnessing the heroic efforts of local communities and neighbourly connections. The global social work statement of ethical principles of social work refers to social justice, human rights, collective responsibility and respect for diversities (IFSW, 2018). One assumes it is not necessary to teach kindness. I hear about the amazing work of third sector organisations and community groups with people from Black, Asian and minority groups, especially since the George Floyd murder (Hill et al, 2020). People tell us in statutory services that they would like more kindness. I have added the word to my leadership tool kit and remind myself daily that it is most important to be a kind leader and to model this value in my work.

We say his name, George Floyd.

We feel unfathomable pain.

In this time when our hearts grieve and our world feels broken, we must stand strong.

We must take action.

To move forward.

Building a society that has zero tolerance for prejudice.

A better word that upholds human decency, equality, kindness and love.

A place where all people are treated the same and with the utmost level of care.

We understand the work is hard and the road ahead will be long.

We embrace our responsibility to not only create a workplace, but a healthy way of life that honours, respects and champions all

(Black Lives Matter, 2020)

Ferlazzo (2020) reminds us that '*kindness did not save George Floyd's life*' and warns against the danger of packaging kindness, mindfulness and resilience into '*glitzy professional-development sessions*'. There is an inherent risk of '*making acts of kindness transactional events rather than natural and expected occurrences*'. He writes about kindness initiatives in school curricula that collapse the value of practising kindness into packages.

From my own experience, I still feel the shock in my body when I recall the day I went out of my house to do my daily exercise. Two white women swore and spat at me. I can only assume this is because I am Chinese and the Chinese were being blamed for the coronavirus. I felt disempowered; I felt discriminated against; I felt wounded.

This wounding, like the death of George Floyd, should serve as a reminder that '*while kindness does matter, our individual and collective humanity matters most*' (Ferlazzo, 2020).

Professional curiosity has become a priority recommendation for safeguarding adults reviews and domestic homicide reviews, often following tragic deaths. Social workers (and other professionals) are told we are not curious enough, we do not look beyond the surface and ask questions which really matter.

We know that children are instinctively curious, until they are discouraged and stopped from asking questions. For professional curiosity to be nurtured and applied in social work practice, leaders have to put in place 'enablers' to create the conditions for cultures of curiosity to develop and grow in their organisations. Thacker et al (2020) highlight the key areas – time and capacity, structure and working practices, supervision and support, open culture, among others – that strategic leaders could focus on to develop the conditions for professional curiosity to flourish.

The Department of Health and Social Care (2020) ethical framework for adult social care during the Covid-19 crisis draws attention to the importance of being able to respond to and adapt to change – a key attribute of a professionally curious person.

One year on

On 16 March 2021, one year on from the first lockdown, we celebrated World Social Work Day with a remote 'banquet for the super heroes' event. Taking the theme from the BBC Great Christmas Menu where celebrity chefs prepared a banquet for key workers, I invited my social workers to work in small groups and come up with a three-course banquet fit for our hard-working staff. I could not believe how seriously they all took to their task and came up with the most creative menus. I had a panel of judges made up of 'foodie' social workers, headed by the chef of our local soup kitchen. We had so much fun. This was also a memorable World Social Work Day for different reasons from the day in 2020.

One year on, I have been running remote reflective space sessions with social workers across different adult social care service areas, something which would have been practically more difficult in the past, as they work in different physical offices. It lifts my heart when I see social workers smiling on the screen at the end of an intensely reflective time. I was able to join a group of British Association of Social Workers (BASW) staff and volunteer coaches in a remote reflective practice session recently. We were asked to find an object during our break which says something about being reflective. I chose this beautiful, curious piece of white stone with holes, which I found in one of my mindful walks. It speaks to me about being attentive enough to look and find and stop to pick it up and being curious enough to ask further questions. I discovered that the holes are made by piddocks and I have been learning a lot since I picked up that first stone. Piddocks are bivalves – their specially adapted shells are edged with fine teeth which they use to excavate burrows in rocks. They are also known as angel wings, which I think is lovely, because of the shape when their shell is opened out. The wonderful thing is that every piece of piddock art is unique – I have several treasured pieces as proof of their handiwork (see Figure 12.1).

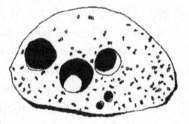

Figure 12.1 An example of a piddock

Many remote working experiences with my own staff and with the wider social work workforce have demonstrated to me that time and time again, and no more so than during the Covid-19 pandemic, the social work profession has demonstrated its capacity to transform crises into better futures.

Where am I now?

So, where am I now as a social worker, belonging to this amazing profession I am still immensely proud of and passionate about? As I am writing about this, the strong visual image of my first team room and the family of social workers I belonged to came back to me. This old-fashioned building no longer exists in Oxford city centre, but the old-fashioned sense of looking out for each other has come back to me with increased energy and purpose.

When I started as a young social worker, I believed in working hard and being loyal to the local authority which employed me to work with the residents of their area. That was my limited 'reach' and I tried to make every small difference count. As I moved to more senior and strategic positions, I started to widen my 'reach' to partnership work outside of my organisation and made allies with so many other professionals. Thirty plus years later, I now want to widen and increase my 'reach' even more. It is possible to go beyond the constraints of physical distance if I take the time to be mindful of and attend to the whole community of the social work profession. I am now more enabled and empowered to bring all aspects of my whole self to my unique role in this profession – my cultural self, my knowledge self, my mindful self, my artful self and my spiritual self. Tao reminds us to 'keep balance between yin and yang, action and thought, self and other ... To be a wise leader in the outer life, one must be a wise leader in the inner life' (Tsai, 2012). Dreher (1996) contended that a leader is one who realises that we have the greatest natural resources in our hearts and minds and those who surround us.

In my 'spare' time, I work as a volunteer coach for the BASW Professional Support Services and as a volunteer spiritual accompanier for our diocese. I took inspiration from Nouwen, a Catholic priest and much-loved spiritual guide, who worked for many years with people with learning disabilities in the L'Arche community (L'Arche in the UK, 2017). I believe leaders must be willing to go beyond their professional roles and leave themselves open as fellow human beings with the same vulnerabilities and wounds as those they serve. In other words, we heal from our wounds. As Nouwen (1979) suggested, it is in common searches and shared risks that we give birth to new ideas and see new visions and new roads ahead.

I am now more ready to take the risk of bringing more of my whole self to my work. Before the pandemic, I never had enough courage or opportunity to bring the artist side of me to my work. Even if I had a sudden inspiration about a piece of art or music which helps to communicate an important message to my staff, I couldn't do anything quickly if I had not included it in my preparation. On a remote platform, I can be more spontaneous and creative. I can quickly find what I need on Google images and screenshare with my staff.

Visual metaphors can be used to help social workers to consider their response to stress and trauma. The practice supervisor development programme (Research in Practice, 2020) offers useful tools to promote discussion about working in challenging circumstances, to use different check-in methods to circumvent the tendency to ask 'how are you?' and get the reply 'I am fine'.

The challenge for the social work leader is to model what it means to be a caring organisation and to be putting relationships at the very heart of what we do 'with' people we serve and 'with' our staff, showing appreciation and working 'with' them. Treisman (2018) refers to '*a fore fronting of self-care, wellbeing and wellness of staff*' which is '*meaningfully infused throughout the organisation*'.

I will end with bringing my spiritual self to join with my mindful self. The Jesuits describe themselves as contemplatives in action and the Society has a long tradition of working with the disadvantaged. Whatever your spirituality, I hope this Jesuit prayer (Pray As You Go, nd) means something to all social workers and social work leaders, who are set with each other '*in the company of healers*'.

'*I ask that today I may be given the grace to cure sometimes, heal often and comfort always.*'

Reflective questions

» Do you think mindfulness is compatible with leadership and management?

» How do you think physical space and environment affects practitioners?

» Do you think there are any well-being advantages to digital connection rather than face-to-face meetings?

References

Black Lives Matter (2020) Rest in Power, Beautiful. [online] Available at: https://blacklivesmatter.com/rest-in-power-beautiful/ (accessed 30 November 2021).

Carter, C (2021) 36 Social Workers of Working Age Died from Covid-19 in 2020, Official Figures Show. *Community Care*, 27 January. [online] Available at: www.communitycare.co.uk/2021/01/27/36-working-age-social-workers-died-covid-19-2020-official-figures-show/ (accessed 30 November 2021).

Department of Health and Social Care (2020) *COVID-19: Ethical Framework for Adult Social Care.* [online] Available at: www.gov.uk/government/publications/covid-19-ethical-framework-for-adult-social-care (accessed 30 November 2021).

Domakin, A (2020) Supporting Remote and Online Supervision During COVID-19. Research in Practice Blog. [online] Available at: www.researchinpractice.org.uk/all/news-views/2020/april/supporting-remote-and-online-supervision-during-covid-19/ (accessed 30 November 2021).

Dreher, D (1996) *The Tao of Personal Leadership.* New York: Harper Collins.

Ferlazzo, L (2020) 'The Problem with Kindness': SEL and the Death of George Floyd. EdWeek. [online] Available at: www.edweek.org/teaching-learning/opinion-the-problem-with-kindness-sel-the-death-of-george-floyd/2020/06 (accessed 30 November 2021)

Hill, E, Tiefenthaler, A, Triebert, C, Jordan, D, Willis, H and Stein, R (2020) How George Floyd Was Killed in Police Custody. *New York Times*, 31 May. [online] Available at: www.nytimes.com/2020/05/31/us/george-floyd-investigation.html (accessed 30 November 2021).

International Federation of Social Work (IFSW) (2018) *Global Social Work Statement of Ethical Principles.* [online] Available at: www.ifsw.org/global-social-work-statement-of-ethical-principles/ (accessed 30 November 2021).

L'Arche in the UK (2017) Henri Nouwen. [online] Available at: www.larche.org.uk/henri-nouwen (accessed 30 November 2021).

Nouwen, H J M (1979) *The Wounded Healer.* Darton, Longman and Todd.

Pray As You Go (nd) Healing Hands Preparation Prayer. [online] Available at: https://pray-as-you-go.org/player/prayer%20tools/2843 (accessed 30 November 2021).

Research in Practice (2020) Resources and Tools for Practice Supervisors. [online] Available at: https://practice-supervisors.rip.org.uk (accessed 30 November 2021).

Samuel, M (2020a) 10 Social Workers Have Died from Covid-19, Official Figures Show. *Community Care*, 12 May. [online] Available at: www.communitycare.co.uk/2020/05/12/10-social-workers-died-covid-19-official-figures-show/ (accessed 30 November 2021).

Samuel, M (2020b) 21 Social Workers Have Died from Covid-19, Show Official Figures. *Community Care*, 28 June. [online] Available at: www.communitycare.co.uk/2020/06/28/21-social-workers-died-covid-19-show-official-figures/ (accessed 30 November 2021).

Stevenson, L (2019) Hotdesking not Compatible with Social Work, 86% of Social Workers Say. *Community Care*. [online] Available at: www.communitycare.co.uk/2019/02/21/hotdesking-compatible-social-work-86-social-workers-say (accessed February 2022).

Thacker, H, Anka, A and Penhale, B (2020) The Importance of Professional Curiosity in Safeguarding Adults. Research in Practice Blog. [online] Available at: www.researchinpractice.org.uk/adults/news-views/2020/december/the-importance-of-professional-curiosity-in-safeguarding-adults/ (accessed 30 November 2021).

Treisman, K (2018) *Becoming a Trauma-Informed Organisation: Practices and Principles.* Churchill Fellowship, supported by the Mental Health Foundation. [online] Available at: www.churchillfellowship.org/ideas-experts/ideas-library/becoming-a-trauma-informed-organisation-practices-and-principles (accessed 11 January 2022).

Tsai, K C (2012) Lead the Way: Tao of Leadership. *Oriental Journal of Social Sciences*, 1: 1.

Turner, A (2020) Social Worker One of Two Employees at Council to Die after Contracting Covid-19. *Community Care*, 31 March. [online] Available at: www.communitycare.co.uk/2020/03/31/social-worker-one-two-employees-council-die-contracting-covid-19/ (accessed 30 November 2021).

Chapter 13 | Can we keep the environment in mind while we adjust to renewed freedoms?

Dr Sandra Engstrom

Introduction

The move to practising social work online brought immense challenges and adaptations, as well as creative thinking and problem solving. Adapting to online work has meant learning to cope with new technologies and ways of building and maintaining professional and personal relationships. This has been an emotional and mental challenge for all. The other side of this coin, however, is that with less travel by students, practitioners and academics, the amount of fossil fuel consumption and other environmental impacts of travelling went through a brief period of decline.

This chapter will look briefly at the environmental impact of social work moving online during the Covid-19 crisis and how we can incorporate this awareness as we move back to a less confined existence. This chapter will offer an opportunity for the reader to reflect on what positive environmental changes happened within their own personal and professional spheres during the Covid-19 pandemic. Although within the UK, at the time of writing, many of the restrictions have eased, it is hoped that some of these sustainable changes can be maintained as we move into an unprecedented era of climate crisis.

Adaptation of the profession

Social workers have played a critical role during this pandemic by supporting service users not only with the needs that brought them to a social worker's attention in the first place, but within the context of Covid-19 which brought additional challenges (Bright, 2020). Social workers have had to cope not only with the risks posed to service users, but the risks that they were facing in their own life. Supporting the range of loss and grief professionally and personally takes a toll on professionals, especially when they are not able to rely on the face-to-face and workplace relationships that are so often essential to the well-being of social workers (Engstrom, 2017).

There is still much to learn about the impact of the pandemic on social work practice and education. What is clear, however, is that social work, along with many other professions, needs to be able to adapt to changing environments while also keeping the core values and skills that are required to support those that need social work involvement (Golightly and Holloway, 2020). The pandemic highlighted and emphasised the inequalities that are already present within society and increased the struggles for those who are most vulnerable and isolated (Abrams and Dettlaff, 2020). The profession is adept and trained to deal with crisis situations – in fact this is often a core standard that social work students have to meet (Scottish Social Services Council, 2019; Bright, 2020). As the global health crisis continues, while also being compounded by the global climate crisis, social workers are going to continue to be called on to respond quickly to those who are most disadvantaged, in contexts of which they may have no prior experience.

The impact of online work and lockdowns on the environment

The pandemic has caused countless severe societal and economic changes to all aspects of our day to day lives. Social and physical distancing directives, national and international travel restrictions and quarantines led to decreases in commuting as the message was given for everyone to work from home, or for others, temporary or permanent loss of employment (Bashir et al, 2020; El Zowalaty et al, 2020). However, the impact of these restricted activities also contributed towards moments of a cleaner environment (Bashir et al, 2020). Although temporary, these positive environmental effects can serve as an example of how certain changes to day to day lives can demonstrate the efficiency and creativity needed to make further positive changes for the natural environment such as a shift to clean energy, which in turn supports human health and well-being.

The Covid-19 pandemic is a global health emergency, but it can also serve as an example of how changes in travel and production can improve air quality and reduce the carbon footprint. During the early months of the pandemic when many major cities were in lockdown, there were significant drops in greenhouse gases (GHGs) in comparison with 2019. Satellite images from NASA indicated that major environmental pollutants decreased by between 20 and 40 per cent (Knowland et al, 2020). Air quality significantly improved as there were lower emissions of air pollutants such as carbon monoxide, nitrous oxide and carbon dioxide in industrial economies (Bashir et al, 2020; Wang and Su, 2020). Specifically, air pollutants in New York dropped by 50 per cent, coal use in China decreased by 40 per cent with an overall 25 per cent reduction in GHG emissions (Guatam, 2020; Saadat et al, 2020; Sarkodie and Owusu,

2021). There were also reports that there was reduced fossil fuel consumption during this time as there was less demand for coal, gasoline and diesel (Bashir et al, 2020; Wang et al, 2020; Sharif et al, 2020).

Water pollution and the impact of sediment churning due to motorboats were also reported to have improved with noticeable changes in the Ganga River in India and in the canals of Venice (Rupani et al, 2020; Saadat et al, 2020). Additionally, the reduction of vehicles on the roads was thought to have decreased the number of wildlife species killed, and the diminished global travel trade is thought to be associated with decreased movement of non-native species and wildlife diseases (Zellmer et al, 2020; Shilling and Waetjen, 2020).

However, although this perhaps provided some emotional relief, the discourse that emerged as a result of reports of animals 'reclaiming' or 'returning' to spaces that are traditionally dominated by humans is one that needs to be treated with caution. As Searle and Turnbull (2020) report, celebrating the pandemic as somehow beneficial to the natural world is dangerous as it fails to acknowledge the complexities in which the pandemic emerged, as well as playing into the anthropocentric view that humans are separate from nature. Additionally, some animals have evolved and adapted to rely on human practices using opportunistic food sources in the form of roadkill or rubbish heaps, while others are reliant on humans for conservation efforts.

This is where developing an eco-social worldview becomes an important process for social workers and those who they work with. No one would claim to have wanted a global pandemic to happen for these relationships to be highlighted, yet there is now a clear chance to use this new or reawakened knowledge to move forward in a more sustainable and environmentally friendly way.

Re-emerging with an eco-social worldview

Social workers are consistently told to think about the person in the environment. This traditionally means the social, political and economic systems that an individual, family or community is connected to. Those who subscribe to the green, eco or environmental social work movement push for the environment to include not only the human and built environment, but the natural and non-human environment (Dominelli, 2012; Besthorn, 2000). Now, more than ever, due to the Covid-19 pandemic as well as the climate crisis that the Intergovernmental Panel on Climate Change (IPCC) (2021) has stated is at *'Code red for humanity'*, social workers have the opportunity to challenge and re-examine the structures of injustices and destruction associated with an anthropocentric worldview that encompasses many workplace systems and practices as well as individual lives.

I have previously written about the importance of embracing an eco-social worldview, which acknowledges the inextricable relationship between humans and all life on earth (Engstrom and Powers, 2021). An eco-social worldview or lens requires us to critically examine and question our current societal structures, practices, policies, routines, values, life-pace and patterns of production and consumption (Engstrom and Powers, 2021). Humans cannot exist without the natural world and it is becoming clearer that we need to re-evaluate our relationship with this and to see ourselves as part of it, as opposed to separate. Eco- or green social work is not new (Besthorn, 2000; Dominelli, 2012), but with our current overlapping and interconnected crises, it is gaining traction as more and more people remember and come to realise that the health and well-being of people is inseparable from the health and well-being of the planet.

During the waves of the pandemic, physical distancing and taking part in collective health-promoting behaviours encouraged us to think beyond ourselves. We had to think collectively about how our behaviours would impact on those around us, whether we knew them or not. This is the same mentality we need to continue moving forward in terms of how we support the natural world that we are a part of and that we need to survive. Connection needs to be an integral part of recovery for those who have had a Covid-19 diagnosis, as well as for all of us who have been distancing from others for so long – connection with others, but also connection with the natural world. The relationship that we have with the natural world has been highlighted as an essential aspect of our health (Alcock et al, 2014) and as so much of social work practice is relationship based, it seems only a natural progression to include the relationship that service users have with the natural world as a component of social work practice.

There is a worry that people will rush to return to 'normal' and consume at the same if not an even greater rate having missed out while lockdown was enforced and due to pressure to restore the economy, and that the benefits of this 'pause' in consumption and movement will be quickly erased. It is essential, especially now with the results of the IPCC (2021) report that social workers reflect on how they can adapt their practice to support societal change to reduce the impact of climate change. Those who are most vulnerable and least responsible are already bearing the brunt of climate change related events, which makes the role of social work in this context even more essential as these individuals, families and communities are already likely to be familiar to social work services. Social workers' understanding of not only the benefits of an eco-social world view but the impact of climate justice on those who are most vulnerable in their practice will hopefully support a green recovery and post-pandemic 'just transition' (Schlosberg and Collins, 2014) that is beneficial for both the human and the non-human natural world.

Conclusion

The early lockdowns during this global pandemic allowed a brief look at what is possible if there is less carbon entering the atmosphere and the ability of humans to think creatively in a crisis. Recovery from the pandemic, as well as from the climate crisis, needs continued reflection and awareness of what systems and structures support the health and well-being of both humans and the natural world. This chapter has briefly explored some of the complexities and nuances of this discussion and the role of social work within it.

Social work must challenge the systems and structures that create natural as well as social problems in the first place. The individuals, families and communities that encounter social work are already victims of climate injustice as well as many additional injustices. Additionally, social workers themselves will also be dealing with the impact of climate change related events if they are not doing so already, which reiterates the IPCC (2021) report that the consequences of climate change are everywhere.

Moments of crisis provide us with opportunities to reflect on our own worldviews and day to day lives and there is no longer any room to deny the trajectory that we are on. Social workers are trained to challenge, think creatively, work holistically and attend to injustices: what is now required is for social workers to include environmental injustices in their remit.

Reflective questions

» What environmentally friendly and sustainable changes have you made either consciously or unconsciously as a result of moving online?

» What changes can you maintain as restrictions are lifted?

» How can you incorporate more of an eco-social worldview into your professional (and personal) routine?

References

Abrams, L S and Dettlaff, A J (2020) Voices from the Frontlines: Social Workers Confront the Covid-19 Pandemic. *Social Work*, 65(3): 302–5.

Alcock, I, White, M P, Wheeler, B W, Fleming, L E and Depledge, M H (2014) Longitudinal Effects on Mental Health of Moving to Greener and Less Green Urban Areas. *Environmental Science and Technology*, 48: 1247–55.

Bashir, M F, Ma, B and Shahzad, L (2020) A Brief Review of Socio-Economic and Environmental Impact of Covid-19. *Air Quality, Atmosphere and Health*, 13: 1403–9.

Besthorn, F H (2000) Toward A Deep-Ecological Social Work: Its Environmental, Spiritual and Political Dimensions. *Spirituality and Social Work Forum*, 7(2): 2–7.

Bright, C L (2020) Social Work in the Age of a Global Pandemic. *Social Work Research*, 44(2): 83–6.

Dominelli, L (2012) *Green Social Work: From Environmental Crises to Environmental Justice*. Cambridge: Polity Press.

El Zowalaty, M E, Young, S G and Järhult, J D (2020) Environmental Impact of the Covid-19 Pandemic: A Lesson for the Future. *Infection Ecology and Epidemiology*, 10: 1–2.

Engstrom, S (2017) Interpersonal Justice: The Importance of Relationships for Child and Family Social Workers. *Journal of Social Work Practice,* 33(1): 41–53.

Engstrom, S and Powers, M (2021) Embracing an Ecosocial Worldview for Climate Justice and Collective Healing. *Journal of Transdisciplinary Peace Praxis*, 3(1): 120–45.

Golightly, M and Holloway, M (2020) Unprecedented Times? Social Work and Society Post Covid-19. *British Journal of Social Work*, 50: 1297–303.

Gautam, S (2020) COVID-19: Air Pollution Remains Low as People Stay at Home. *Air Quality, Atmosphere and Health*, 13: 853–7.

Intergovernmental Panel on Climate Change (IPCC) (2021) *Climate Change 2021: Sixth Assessment Report*. [online] Available at: www.ipcc.ch/assessment-report/ar6/ (accessed 16 January 2022).

Knowland, E K, Keller, C, Ott, L, Pawson, S, Saunders, E, Wales, P and Duncan, B (2020) Local to Global Air Quality Simulations using the NASA GEOS Composition Forecast Model, GEOS-CF. [online] Available at: www.semanticscholar.org/paper/Local-to-Global-Air-Quality-Simulations-using-the-Knowland-Keller/9f64d9ea383109e9a8a60fd0a8097ed11c62637a (accessed 16 January 2022).

Rupani, P F, Nilashi, M, Abumalloh, R A, Asadi, S, Samad S and Wang, S (2020) Coronavirus Pandemic (Covid-19) and its Natural Environmental Impacts. *International Journal of Environmental Science and Technology*, 17: 4655–66.

Saadat, S, Rawtani, D and Hussain, C M (2020) Environmental Perspective of Covid-19. *Science of the Total Environment*, 728: 1–6.

Sarkodie, S A and Owusu, P A (2021) Global Assessment of Environment, Health and Economic Impact of the Novel Coronavirus (Covid-19). *Environment, Development and Sustainability*, 23: 5005–15.

Schlosberg, D and Collins, L B (2014) From Environmental to Climate Justice: Climate Change and the Discourse of Environmental Justice. *WIRE's Climate Change*, 5: 359–74.

Scottish Social Services Council (2019) *Standards in Social Work Education*. Dundee. [online] Available at: https://learn.sssc.uk.com/siswe/uploads/files/SiSWE-and-Ethical-Principles.pdf (accessed 20 January 2022).

Searle, A and Turnbull, J (2020) Resurgent Natures? More-than-human Perspectives on Covid-19. *Dialogues in Human Geography*, 10(2): 291–5.

Sharif, A, Aloui, C and Yarovaya, L (2020) COVID-19 Pandemic, Oil Prices, Stock Market, Geopolitical Risk and Policy Uncertainty Nexus in the U.S. Economy: Fresh Evidence from the Wavelet-based Approach. *International Review of Financial Analysis*, 70: 101496.

Shilling, F and Waetjen, D (2020) *Special Report: Impact of COVID19 on California Traffic Accidents.* California: UC Davis.

Wang, P, Chen, K, Zhu, S, Wang, P and Zhang, H (2020) Severe Air Pollution Events Not Avoided by Reduced Anthropogenic Activities During COVID-19 Outbreak. *Resources, Conservation and Recycling,* 158: 104814.

Wang, Q and Su, M (2020) A Preliminary Assessment of the Impact of COVID-19 on Environment: A Case Study of China. *The Science of the Total Environment,* 728: 138915.

Zellmer, A J, Wood, E M, Surasinghe, T, Putman, B J, Pauly, G B, Magle, S B, Lewis, J S, Kay, C A M and Fidino, M (2020) What Can We Learn from Wildlife Sightings During the Covid-19 Global Shutdown? *Ecosphere,* 11(8): e0321.

Concluding thoughts

Dr Denise Turner and Dr Michael Fanner

When the companion volume to this book, *Social Work and Covid-19: Lessons for Education and Practice* (Turner, 2021) was nearing publication in December 2020, the very first Covid-19 vaccine had only just been administered to the then 91-year-old Margaret Keenan (BBC News, 2020). As this new book goes to press, however, both editors have shared conversations about the side-effects they themselves experienced from the third 'booster' jabs, something which would have been unthinkable less than a year earlier. With the rollout of this vaccine programme, the contributions of the NHS and those educators and practitioners who support it have been illuminated and chapters in this book testify to this. From Craig Harman's inspirational account of training within the St John Ambulance service, through Timothy Kuhn's description of preparing redeployed practitioners, to Henrietta Mbeah-Bankas' discussion of educating the future health workforce, alongside others on medical and practice education, the creativity and commitment of the health response to Covid-19 is clear and unambiguous.

For social work and social care, described by the British Association of Social Workers in 2021 as the 'forgotten frontline' (BASW, 2021), the commitment has nevertheless been as powerful and as demonstrable and chapters in this book give voice to the creative ways in which relationships have been sustained through challenging times. The case studies in Chapter 10, authored by Hilary Woodhead and Natalie Ravenscroft of the National Activity Providers Association, are profoundly poignant in the deep human connections evidenced, as care home staff embraced and at times struggled with new technologies, whereas in Chapter 11, the creative thread is looped through the description of sustaining connection through moving a traditionally arts-based module online. Annie Ho in Chapter 12 takes care to remind those in leadership positions to embrace creativity and remain mindful of their own well-being and that of the staff that they lead, while the next generation of social workers emerge powerfully from Chapter 4, despite the struggles described by the authors during the pandemic and the move to online learning.

As co-editors, it has been a genuine pleasure to work across disciplines and to build understanding of the differences and similarities in the professional experiences described within the book. At times, progress on the book itself has been hindered by impacts from Covid-19, such as increased workloads, or unexpected symptoms following vaccines, but for the most part authors have met deadlines with notable generosity and fortitude. This is particularly impressive considering that all the authors in this book have so many competing demands on their time, from practice-based pressures to those of teaching and learning.

Finally, regardless of professional discipline, the last chapter in this book, written by Dr Sandra Engstrom, invites all of us to use learning from the pandemic as an opportunity to challenge the systems and structures that are threatening to cause irreversible environmental disaster.

As Arundhati Roy (2020) suggests in 'The Pandemic is a Portal' we have a choice moving forward, either to *'choose to walk through it, dragging the carcasses of our prejudice and hatred, our avarice, our data banks and dead ideas, our dead rivers and smoky skies behind us'*. Alternatively, we can *'walk through lightly, with little luggage, ready to imagine another world. And ready to fight for it.'*

With the World Health Organization forecasts of further pandemics in the future and the impacts of climate change related events across the globe, it is perhaps now more vital than ever before that we make the right choice, as Chapter 13 invites. By deploying some of the courage, good practice, curiosity and commitment evidenced by authors in this book and in wider health, social work and social care during the pandemic, we have a sound foundation to begin. This book represents a very modest contribution to moving forwards with collaboration and co-production and as co-editors we are profoundly grateful to all the contributors and to the enduringly patient publisher who made it possible.

References

British Association of Social Work (BASW) (2021) Survey Unveils the Heavy Toll on Social Workers – A 'Forgotten Frontline' – as Restrictions Limit Their Capacity to Safeguard Vulnerable Adults and Children. 28 January. [online] Available at: www.basw.co.uk/media/news/2021/jan/survey-unveils-heavy-toll-social-workers--'forgotten-frontline'--restrictions (accessed 10 January 2022).

BBC News (2020) Covid-19 Vaccine: First Person Receives Pfizer Jab in UK. 8 December. [online] Available at: www.bbc.co.uk/news/uk-55227325 (accessed 3 January 2022).

Roy, A (2020) The Pandemic is a Portal. *Financial Times*, April 3. [online] Available at: www.ft.com/content/10d8f5e8-74eb-11ea-95fe-fcd274e920ca (accessed 11 January 2022).

Turner, D (ed) (2021) *Social Work and Covid-19: Lessons for Education and Practice.* St Albans: Critical Publishing.

Index